Health Care for ADOLESCENTS

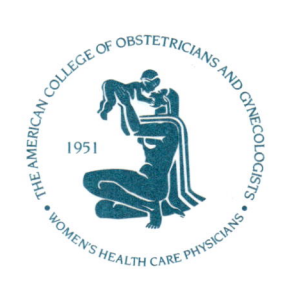

The American College of
Obstetricians and Gynecologists

Women's Health Care Physicians

409 12th Street, SW
PO Box 96920
Washington, DC 20090-6920

Health Care for Adolescents was developed by the ACOG Committee on Adolescent Health Care. Past and present committee members who have contributed to the development of this document include: Trina M. Anglin, MD; Sylvester R. Braithwaite, MD; Richard R. Brookman, MD; Jacqueline E. Darroch, PhD; Ann J. Davis, MD; Robert J. Fagnant, MD; S. Paige Hertweck, MD; Melisa M. Holmes, MD; Elisabeth H. Quint, MD; and Jeannette South-Paul, MD.

The information in *Health Care for Adolescents* should not be viewed as a body of rigid rules. The guidelines are general and intended to be adapted to many different stituations, taking into account the needs and resources particular to the locality, the institution, or the type of practice. Variations and innovations that improve the quality of patient care are to be encouraged rather than restricted.

Library of Congress Cataloging-in-Publication Data

Health care for adolescents / The American College of Obstetricians and Gynecologists, Women's Health Care Physicians.
    p. ; cm.
Includes bibliographical references and index.
ISBN 0-915473-94-1
1. Adolescent medicine. 2. Teenage girls—Health and hygiene.
3. Adolescent gynecology.   I. American College of Obstetricians and Gynecologists. Women's Health Care Physicians.
[DNLM: 1. Adolescent Health Services. 2. Eating Disorders
—prevention & control—Adolescence. 3. Parent-Child Relations.
4. Sexually Transmitted Diseases—prevention & control—Adolescence. 5. Suicide—prevention & control—Adolescence.
  WA 330 H434 2003]
  RJ550.H425 2003
  613'.04243—dc21
                                                                2002153043

Copyright © 2003 by the American College of Obstetricians and Gynecologists, 409 12th Street, SW, PO Box 96920, Washington, DC 20090-6920. All rights reserved. No part of this publication may be reproduced, stored in a retrieval system, or transmitted, in any form or by any means electronic, mechanical, photocopying, recording, or otherwise, without prior written permission from the publisher.

Copies of *Health Care for Adolescents* can be ordered through the ACOG Distribution Center by calling toll free 800-762-2264. Orders also can be placed from the ACOG web site at www.acog.org or sales.acog.org.

12345/76543

Contents

Preface	v
Acknowledgments	vi
Primary and Preventive Health Care for Female Adolescents	1
Confidentiality in Adolescent Health Care	25
Oral Contraceptives for Adolescents: Benefits and Safety	37
Condom Availability for Adolescents	53
Adolescents' Right to Refuse Long-term Contraceptives	63
Screening for Chlamydia and Gonorrhea in Adolescents	69
Eating Disorders	81
Preventing Adolescent Suicide	95
Appendix A	107
Appendix B	109
Index	111

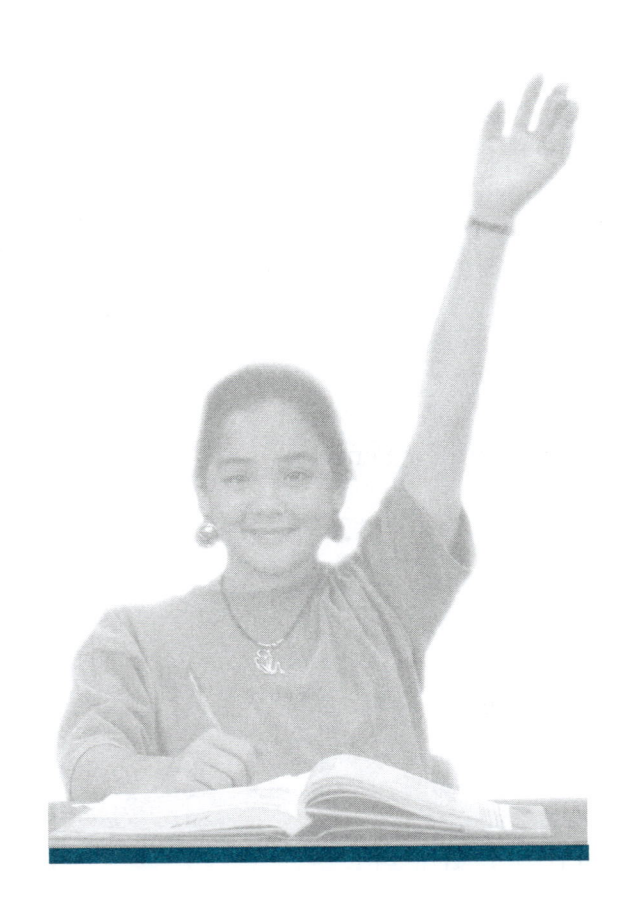

Preface

Adolescence is a time of psychosocial, cognitive, and physical development as young people make the transition from childhood to adulthood. For many adolescents, this transition is relatively smooth, but for others, it can be a time of difficulty. Guidance from a physician for the adolescent and her parents, as well as the provision of needed health screening and care, can greatly facilitate adolescents' healthy transition to adulthood.

The American College of Obstetricians and Gynecologists (ACOG) believes that health care professionals have an obligation to provide the best possible care to respond to the needs of their adolescent patients. This care should, at a minimum, include primary and preventive care and comprehensive reproductive health services, such as sexuality education, counseling, mental health assessment, diagnosis and treatment regarding pubertal development, access to contraceptives and abortion, pregnancy-related care, prenatal and delivery care, and diagnosis and treatment of sexually transmitted diseases (see Appendix A and Appendix B).*

Health Care for Adolescents is designed to provide the information necessary for the provision of health services to adolescent patients in a comprehensive fashion. It contains new information in addition to the Educational Bulletins and Committee Opinions issued by the Committee on Adolescent Health Care of the American College of Obstetricians and Gynecologists as of December 31, 2002. The documents have been updated and compiled into one volume for ease of use and reference. Previous separate Educational Bulletins and Committee Opinions encompassed in this volume are listed as follows:

Adolescents' Right to Refuse Long-Term Contraceptives (CO No. 139, June 1994)

Condom Availability for Adolescents (CO No. 154, April 1995)

Confidentiality in Adolescent Health Care (EB No. 249, August 1998)

Oral Contraceptives for Adolescents: Benefits and Safety (EB NO. 256, December 1999)

Prevention of Adolescent Suicide (CO No. 190, October 1997)

Primary and Preventive Health Care for Female Adolescents (EB No. 254, November 1999)

ACOG Committee on Adolescent Health Care

---

*American College of Obstetricians and Gynecologists. Guidelines for women's health care. 2nd ed. Washington, DC: ACOG; 2002.

Acknowledgments

The ACOG Committee on Adolescent Health Care is grateful for the contribution and guidance provided by Lisa Smith Goldstein, MS, Director, Adolescent Health Care, without whose research, writing, and editing the development of this document would not have been possible. The committee would also like to thank Estherann Grace, MD, Associate Clinical Professor, Pediatrics, Harvard Medical School, for her assistance in the development of the chapter on eating disorders. Finally, the Committee on Adolescent Health Care wishes to thank Luella Klein, MD, Vice President, Women's Health Issues; Janet Chapin, RN, MPH, Director, Women's Health Issues; and Noriko Cruz, ACOG intern.

For additional information about the Committee on Adolescent Health Care, please contact Lisa Smith Goldstein, MS, Director, Adolescent Health Care, ACOG, PO Box 96920, Washington, DC 20090-6920; Tel: (202) 863-2497; e-mail: adolhlth@acog.org.

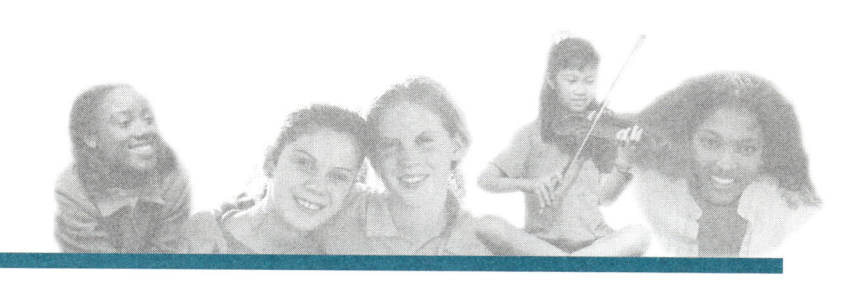

Primary and Preventive Health Care for Female Adolescents

Key points

- The primary health risks to adolescents are behavioral, such as a sedentary lifestyle, poor diet, smoking, alcohol and drug use, driving under the influence of drugs or alcohol, early initiation of sexual activity, and poor use of contraception.

- Adolescent girls should first visit an obstetrician–gynecologist between ages 13 and 15 years, followed by annual visits. Care should be delivered according to the individual's stage of physical, sexual, psychologic, and cognitive development.

- The initial visit generally does not include a pelvic examination. A pelvic examination should be performed when indicated by the medical history (eg, pubertal aberrancy, abnormal bleeding, or abdominal or pelvic pain). If the patient has had sexual intercourse, screening for sexually transmitted diseases is appropriate, and the patient should have her first Pap test no later than 3 years after first intercourse.

- Annual visits provide opportunities to discuss normal development; receive screening for physical, emotional, and behavioral conditions; and obtain immunizations. A physical examination is not required at every visit, but should be included at least once during early, middle, and late adolescence.

- Periodic health guidance is critical for both adolescents and their parents and caregivers. Parents and caregivers should receive guidance at least once during their child's early, middle, and late adolescence; adolescents should receive guidance annually with an emphasis on health promotion and risk reduction strategies.

- All adolescents should be screened annually for hypertension, eating disorders, tobacco use, alcohol and drug use, sexual activity, depression, abuse, and school performance. Those at risk for hyperlipidemia and adult coronary health disease also should have their cholesterol levels checked.

- All sexually active adolescents should be screened annually for gonorrhea and chlamydia. If they are at high risk, they also should be screened for syphilis.

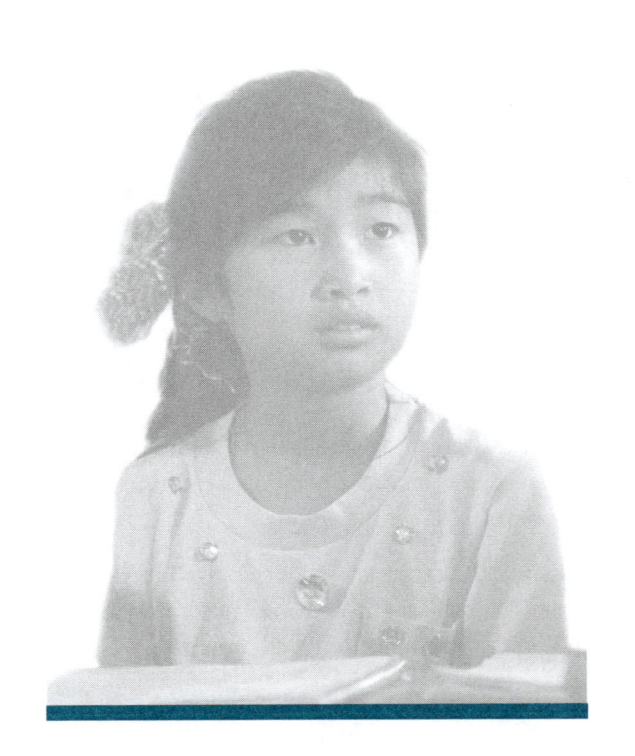

Adolescence is a time of transition from childhood to adulthood and is marked by a number of developmental milestones. For many, this transition is relatively smooth; for others, however, it may be a time of difficulty. Adolescent girls, in particular, are confronted with numerous challenges, and the decisions they make can have both short- and long-term consequences for their health and well-being. The primary health risks to adolescents are no longer the traditional medical causes of illness; rather, they are behavioral. These risks include a sedentary lifestyle, poor nutritional habits, cigarette smoking, alcohol and illicit drug use, driving under the influence of alcohol, early initiation of sexual activity, and poor use of contraception. Most adolescents will engage in one of these unhealthy and risky behaviors, and data from the *2001 Youth Risk Behavior Surveillance Report* indicate that many will begin exhibiting one of these risky behaviors by age 13 years (1). Furthermore, approximately three quarters of all deaths among adolescents and young adults (aged 15–24 years) in 2000 resulted from three preventable causes: 1) unintentional injuries (including motor vehicle crashes) (45%), 2) homicide (16%), or 3) suicide (13%) (2). Guidance from a physician can greatly facilitate a young girl's healthy transition to adulthood. Physicians can provide preventive guidance to both parents and adolescents. They can screen for health-risk behaviors and diseases and can either provide or refer patients for the necessary immunizations against infectious diseases. This chapter will address female adolescent development and primary and preventive health care intervention, including timing of health care visits, health guidance for parents and adolescents, screening, and immunization.

Female Adolescent Development

The delivery of preventive services to adolescents differs from the delivery of preventive services to adults. Although diseases and behaviors among adolescents and adults may or may not be similar, an adolescent's unique developmental stage dictates the framing of preventive services. Furthermore, not all adolescents of the same age are at the same stage of development, thus necessitating further examination of the adolescent's physical, sexual, psychosocial, and cognitive development. Understanding

...an adolescent's unique developmental stage dictates the framing of preventive services.

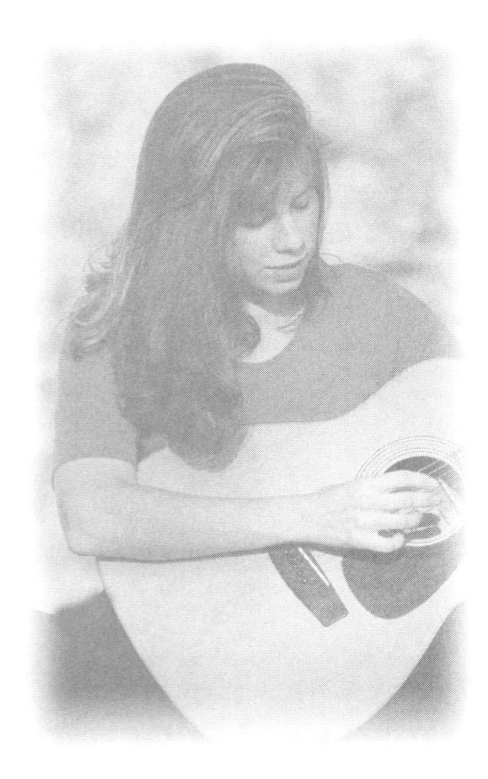

the milestones and developmental stages of adolescence is beneficial to obstetrician–gynecologists treating adolescents.

SEXUAL DEVELOPMENT

Thelarche, or breast budding, the first sign of secondary sexual development in most adolescent females, occurs for most young girls in North America at age 8–10 years. Production of low amounts of estrogen stimulates long bone growth, with a peak height growth of 9 cm per year. When higher levels of estrogen are produced, breast development progresses, long bone growth decelerates, and the epiphyses close. Menarche occurs during this deceleration phase. On average, the first menses occurs between age 12–13 years, with regular ovulation established by approximately 20 cycles later. The average duration of puberty is 4 years, with a range of 1.5 years to 8 years. Data from a large-scale cross-sectional study indicate that at every age and for the development of each pubertal characteristic, African-American girls are more advanced than white girls (3). Based on these data, the Lawson Wilkins Pediatric Endocrine Society recommended new guidelines for the evaluation of premature development. These guidelines state that pubic hair or breast development requires evaluation only when it occurs before age 7 years in non-African-American girls and before age 6 years in African-American girls. These guidelines are reasonable only in the absence of symptoms, such as rapid growth, new central nervous system-related findings, or behavior-based factors (4). If there is any uncertainty, an evaluation should be performed and referrals made, as appropriate. In addition, tempo and sequence aberrancies during an otherwise established pubertal process should be included for evaluation of delayed or precocious sexual development.

PSYCHOSOCIAL AND COGNITIVE DEVELOPMENT

Adolescence is a prolonged period of transition during which a young person's expanding horizons, self-discovery, and quest for independence lead to the formation of a separate and distinct identity (5). It is particularly challenging because the processes of physical, psychologic, and cognitive development occur on separate tracks, with different timetables, which rarely are synchronous. Thus, an obstetrician–gynecologist often will encounter a young girl who has matured physically but has not accomplished important psychologic and cognitive developmental tasks that will allow her to: 1) understand the consequences of present behaviors on future health outcomes and make crucial decisions about the future, 2) understand the saliency of risks and internalize those risks, and 3) form and maintain stable and healthy relationships while evolving and learning to communicate a value system of her own.

The adolescent often believes that she is different from others and, therefore, not liable to the risks that threaten her peers. Although on an intellectual level these risks may be well understood, adolescent behaviors tend to reflect an assumption of invulnerability. Such egocentrism generally is outgrown with continuing cognitive development and a young person's perception of "self" relative to "others." As the girl progresses through adolescence, she becomes increasingly capable, both cognitively and emotionally, of comprehending abstract ideas, relating present actions to future outcomes, and understanding the consequences of her own behaviors. Thus, the clinical approach to counseling a younger adolescent will differ from the approach taken with an older adolescent or an adult.

Timing of Health Care Visits

INITIAL VISIT

Obstetrician–gynecologists frequently are asked by adult patients at what age their adolescent daughters should visit an obstetrician–gynecologist. The first visit to the obstetrician–gynecologist for health guidance, screening, and the provision of preventive health care services should take place between the ages of 13 and 15 years (6). Because the obstetrician–gynecologist can function as either a primary care physician or a consultant specialist, it is important to determine whether the adolescent patient has a primary care provider. If so, a collaborative relationship between physicians should be established.

The exact timing and scope of the initial visit to the obstetrician–gynecologist will depend on the individual girl and her physical and emotional development. Parents and adolescent females should be reassured that the initial visit at this age serves primarily to establish rapport between the obstetrician–gynecologist and the young woman and generally does not include a pelvic examination. This visit is an ideal opportunity to discuss with both parents and adolescents normal adolescent development and other concerns related to adolescence.

To provide optimum health care, physicians should discuss issues of confidentiality with both the adolescent and her parent(s). (See "Confidentiality in Adolescent Health Care" chapter for more on confidentiality issues). Confidentiality frequently is identified as a major obstacle to the delivery of health care services to adolescents. To overcome this barrier, physicians should initiate discussion of this topic, advise the adolescent patient and her parent(s) of relevant state and local statutes, and stress the importance of open communication between all parties.

The provision of additional services beyond guidance and screening should be based on the information obtained at this initial visit. A pelvic examination should be performed when indicated by the medical history (eg, pubertal aberrancy, abnormal bleeding, or abdominal or pelvic pain). If the patient has had sexual intercourse, screening for sexually transmitted diseases (STDs) is appropriate, and the patient should have her first Pap test no later than 3 years after first intercourse.

Annual Visits

Because the potential for unhealthy behaviors and poor health outcomes is significant during adolescence, the initial consultation visit should be followed by annual preventive health care visits. Annual visits contribute to the formation of a trusting relationship between the adolescent patient and her physician. This, in turn, eases the disclosure of high-risk behaviors and facilitates the early diagnosis of physical and emotional disorders. Such visits also enhance the physician's credibility as a caring adult and, therefore, lend weight to recommendations that promote good health. Finally, annual visits enable the adolescent to assume increasingly greater responsibility for her health and well-being.

The proactive, annual preventive health care visit should focus on health guidance for both the patient and parent(s), including a discussion of normal adolescent development; screening for physical, emotional, and behavioral conditions; and immunizations. Primary and preventive health care for adolescents should be based on the guidelines summarized in this chapter. Physicians should tailor the content of their health guidance, screening, and level of parental involvement to the unique requirements of each patient. A physical examination is not required at every visit, but should be performed at least once during early adolescence (ages 12–14 years), middle adolescence (ages 15–17 years), and late adolescence (ages 18–21 years). A pelvic examination should be performed when indicated by the medical history (eg, pubertal aberrancy, abnormal bleeding, or abdominal or pelvic pain). If the patient has had sexual intercourse, screening for STDs is appropriate and the patient should have her first Pap test no later than 3 years after first intercourse.

To help adolescents navigate the transition from childhood to adulthood, a number of organizations have formulated guidelines for adolescent preventive health care services. Guidelines for Adolescent Preventive Services (GAPS), developed for the American Medical Association by a national group of experts, including representatives from the American College of Obstetricians and Gynecologists, form the basis of the following recommendations (7). These recommendations are grouped into three categories: 1) health guidance for both parents and adolescents, 2) screening, and 3) immunization.

Health Guidance

Periodic health guidance for parents and adolescents is a critical component of primary and preventive health care. This is different from obtaining the past medical history because it involves the counseling and discussion component of the health care visit. Health guidance provides an opportunity for physicians, adolescent patients, and their parents to address current and potential health care needs.

Health guidance provides an opportunity for physicians, adolescent patients, and their parents to address current and potential health care needs.

FOR THE PARENTS

Parents and other adult caregivers should receive health guidance at least once during their child's early adolescence, once during middle adolescence, and preferably once during late adolescence. Such guidance can be provided either concurrent to the adolescent's visit or as a separate visit. Health guidance for parents includes information about the following areas:

- Normal adolescent development, including information about physical, sexual, and emotional development
- Signs and symptoms of common diseases and morbidities in adolescents, including depression and emotional distress, to alert parents to the potential health risks facing their children
- Physical and psychosocial benefits gained from participation in sports and other supervised extracurricular activities
- Parenting behaviors that promote healthy adolescent adjustments, including:
  - Allowing increased autonomy and responsibility
  - Anticipating challenges to parental authority
  - Jointly establishing family rules and the consequences for breaking them and enforcing those rules and consequences
  - Enhancing self-esteem with praise and recognition of positive behaviors and achievements
  - Minimizing criticism
  - Respecting privacy
  - Spending time with the adolescent
- Ways to minimize potentially harmful behaviors by:
  - Monitoring and managing the adolescent's use of motor vehicles
  - Avoiding weapons in the home or ensuring that adolescents follow weapon safety procedures
  - Removing weapons and potentially lethal medications from the home of a suicidal adolescent
  - Monitoring the adolescent's social and recreational activities, including tobacco, alcohol, and drug use and sexual behavior, particularly in early and middle adolescence
  - Remaining involved in the adolescent's use of her free time, including television and Internet usage, particularly in early and middle adolescence
  - Monitoring peer relationships

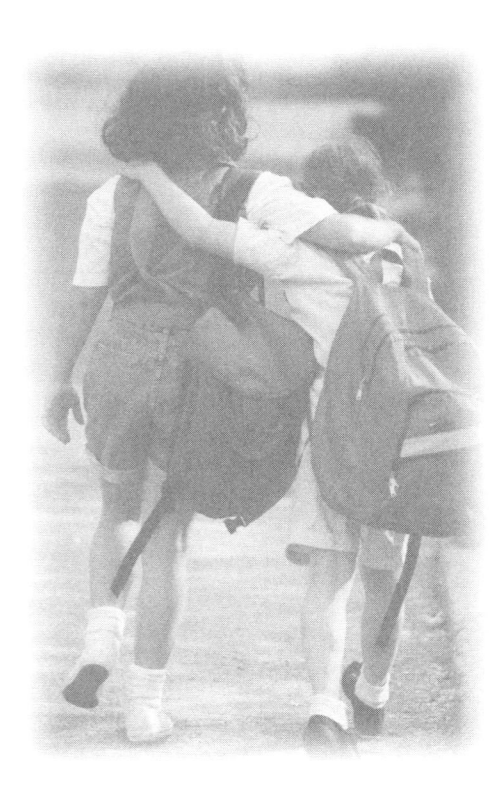

—Recognizing the adolescent's vulnerability in unequal relationships, such as those with older partners or when the partner is in a position of relative authority over the adolescent (8)

—Encouraging the regular use of sunscreen

Additionally, it is important for parents to recognize the influential role of the media, particularly as a source of sexual information for adolescents. At an age when many girls experience a decrease in their self-esteem (9), youth-oriented magazines reinforce sexual stereotypes, emphasize physical appearances, and advise girls on attracting adolescent males. In these popular publications, sexually explicit materials and abstinence-only messages are included together, and little or no information is provided to help readers make healthy, safe, and responsible decisions. Such materials further contribute to the difficult choices that increasingly younger girls are forced to consider. Recognition of these sources of information can help both parents and physicians in their efforts to ensure the health of adolescent girls.

For the Adolescent

Adolescents should receive annual health guidance to promote a better understanding of their physical, psychosocial, and psychosexual development. Such guidance should emphasize health promotion and risk reduction strategies. The importance of becoming actively involved in decisions regarding their own health care also should be stressed.

Screening provides an excellent opportunity to counsel adolescents about healthy lifestyles. Because of concerns regarding mutual trust, issues of confidentiality, and individual comfort levels when discussing sensitive topics, eliciting an accurate response from an adolescent can be difficult. Often, repeated questioning over time is necessary to obtain accurate and complete information.

Health guidance for the adolescent should address diet and physical activity, healthy sexual lifestyle, and injury prevention, as follows:

- Dietary habits, including ways to achieve a healthy diet and safe weight management
- The benefits of physical activity and encouragement to engage regularly in safe physical activities
- Responsible, consensual sexual behavior, including counseling on:
    —Abstinence from sexual intercourse and information that this method is the most effective way to prevent pregnancy and STDs, including human immunodeficiency virus (HIV) infection
    —Responsible sexual behavior for adolescents who are not currently sexually active and for those who are using birth control and condoms appropriately
    —The effectiveness of latex condoms in reducing the risk of pregnancy and STDs, including HIV infection

—Human immunodeficiency virus transmission and the dangers of the disease

—Reducing the risk of sexual victimization and acquaintance rape, including the role of alcohol and other drugs

—Information on emergency contraception, including the 24-hour, national toll-free hotline number 1-888-NOT-2-LATE

- Prevention of injuries, including:

    —Avoiding the use of alcohol or other substances

    —Avoiding driving a motor vehicle or other recreational vehicle if the adolescent has consumed alcohol or other substances

    —Avoiding riding in a car or other recreational vehicle if the driver has consumed alcohol or other substances

    —Encouraging adolescents and their parents to develop agreements for picking-up adolescents who have consumed alcohol or other substances

    —Using safety devices, including seat belts, motorcycle and bicycle helmets, and appropriate athletic protective devices

    —Using nonviolent conflict resolution

    —Avoiding the use of weapons or promoting weapon safety

    —Promoting appropriate physical conditioning before exercise

Screening

BLOOD PRESSURE

All adolescents should be screened annually for hypertension according to the protocol developed by the National Heart, Lung, and Blood Institute Task Force on High Blood Pressure in Children and Adolescents (10). Although the incidence of hypertension in adolescence is low, early detection of elevated blood pressure and evaluation for hypertension risk factors may prevent later cardiovascular diseases.

Body size is the single most important determinant of blood pressure in children and adolescents (10). By accounting for different levels of growth when evaluating blood pressure, a more precise classification can be made, thus avoiding misclassification of those adolescents at the extremes for normal growth (Fig. 1). Listed in Box 1 are steps for assessing classification of blood pressure.

The National Heart, Lung, and Blood Institute's task force has defined normal blood pressure as systolic blood pressure and diastolic blood pressure levels below the 90th percentile for age and sex. High-normal blood pressure is average systolic blood pressure or diastolic blood pressure levels greater than or equal to the 90th percentile, but below the 95th percentile. Hypertension in adolescence is defined as average systolic or diastolic blood

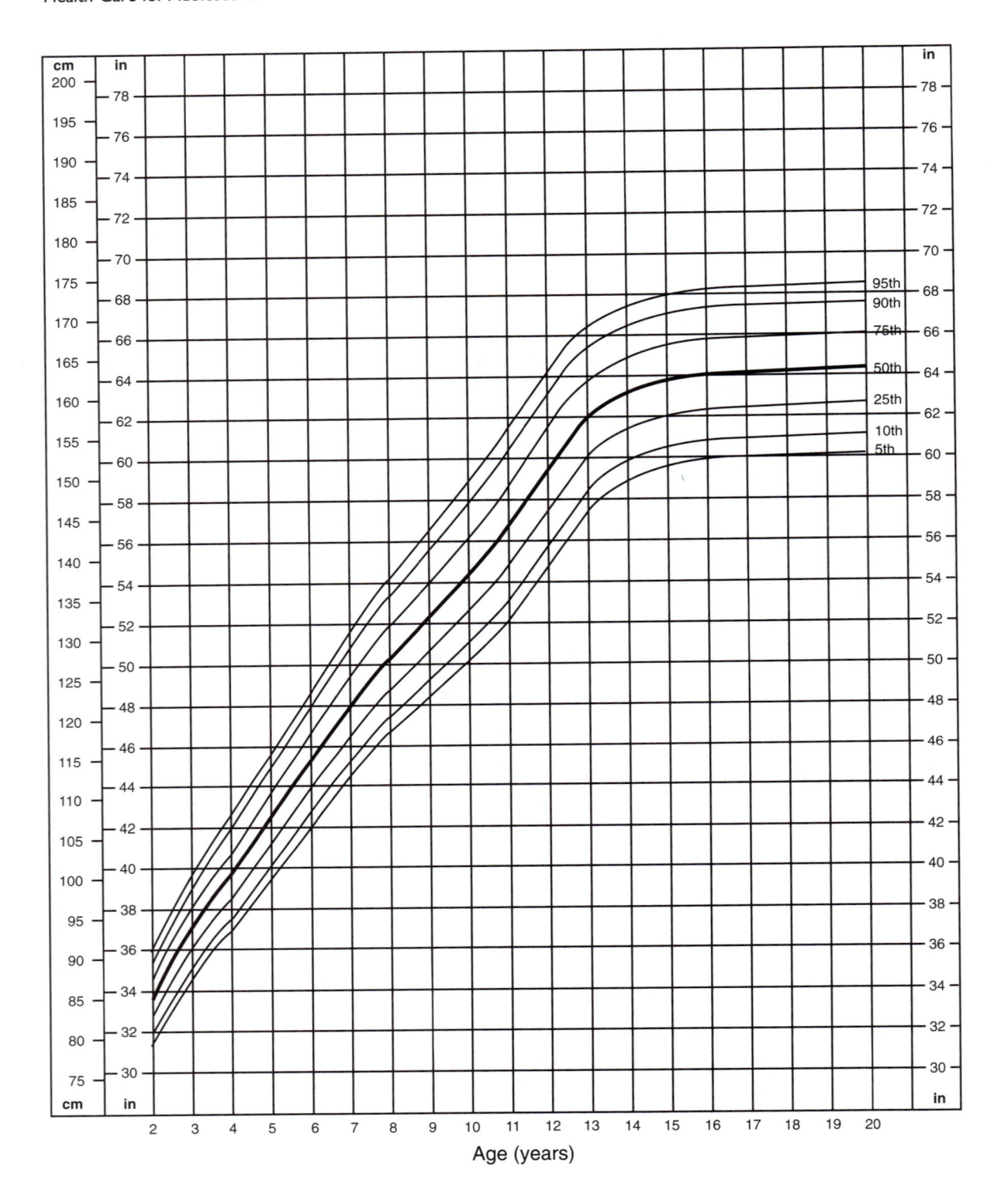

Fig. 1. Girls' stature by age percentiles. (Developed by the National Center for Health Statistics in collaboration with the National Center for Chronic Disease Prevention and Health Promotion [2000].)

pressure levels greater than or equal to the 95th percentile for age and sex measured on at least three separate occasions.

In adolescents with either systolic blood pressure or diastolic blood pressure levels at or above the 90th percentile for age (Fig. 2A), blood pressure measurements should be repeated at three different times within 1 month, under similar physical conditions, to confirm baseline value. After a baseline value has been confirmed, adolescents with baseline blood pressure values greater than the 95th percentile for age (Fig. 2B) should undergo a complete biomedical evaluation to establish treatment options. Adolescents with blood pressure values between the 90th and 95th percentiles should be assessed for predisposing factors, such as obesity, and their blood pressure should be checked every 6 months.

CHOLESTEROL

To determine their risk of developing hyperlipidemia and adult coronary heart disease, adolescents should be screened by history using the following guidelines. Selected adolescents should undergo lipid testing according to the protocol developed by the Expert Panel on Blood Cholesterol in Children and Adolescents (11):

- Adolescents whose parents have a serum cholesterol level greater than 240 mg/dL should be screened for total blood cholesterol (nonfasting) at least once.
- Adolescents with either an unknown family history or multiple risk factors for future cardiovascular disease (eg, smoking, hypertension, obesity, diabetes mellitus, excessive consumption of dietary saturated fats and cholesterol) may be screened for total serum cholesterol level (nonfasting) at least once at the discretion of the physician.

Box 1. Steps for Assessing Classification of Blood Pressure

1. Use the standard height chart to determine the height percentile (see Fig. 1).
2. Measure the adolescent's blood pressure. Record systolic and diastolic blood pressure levels.
3. Find the adolescent's age on the right side of the 90th percentile chart for diastolic blood pressure (see Fig. 2). Follow the age line horizontally across the chart to the intersection of the line for the height percentile (vertical line).
4. Move up or down the height percentile line to the intersection of measured blood pressure.

Result on 90th Percentile Chart

- If you move down on the height percentile line, blood pressure is normal. Repeat steps 3 and 4 on the chart for 90th percentile systolic blood pressure.
- If you move up on the height percentile line, you must repeat steps 3 and 4 on the chart for 95th percentile diastolic blood pressure.

Result on 95th Percentile Chart

- If you move down on the height percentile line, blood pressure is high-normal. Repeat steps 3 and 4 on the chart for 95th percentile systolic blood pressure.
- If you move up on the height percentile line, hypertension* is indicated. Repeat steps 3 and 4 on the chart for 95th percentile systolic blood pressure.

---

*Note that hypertension is diagnosed after three consecutive blood pressure readings above the 95th percentile on three separate occasions.

Modified from National High Blood Pressure Education Program. Update on the Task Force Report (1987) on High Blood Pressure in Children and Adolescents: a working group report from the National High Blood Pressure Education Program. National Institutes of Health, National Heart, Lung, and Blood Institute. Bethesda, MD: National High Blood Pressure Education Program, 1996; NIH publication no. 96-3790.

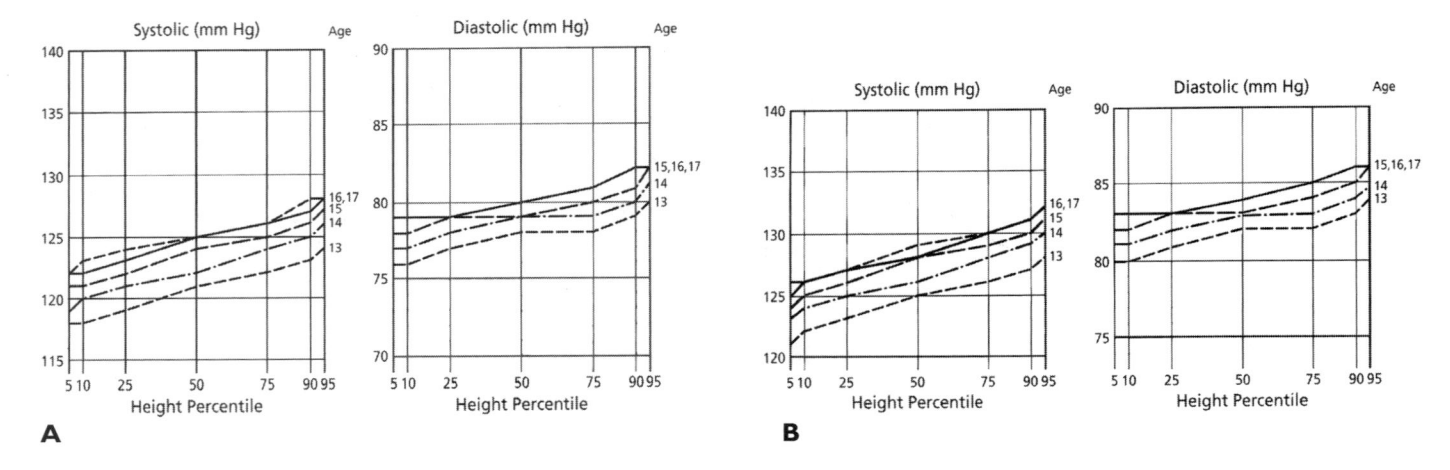

Fig. 2. Systolic and diastolic blood pressure by height and age for girls in the 90th percentile (**A**) and girls in the 95th percentile (**B**). (Modified from National High Blood Pressure Education Program. Update on the Task Force Report [1987] on High Blood Pressure in Children and Adolescents: a working group report from the National High Blood Pressure Education Program. National Institutes of Health, National Heart, Lung and Blood Institute. Bethesda [MD]: National High Blood Pressure Education Program; 1996. NIH publication no. 96-3790.)

- In adolescents with blood cholesterol values less than 170 mg/dL, the test should be repeated in 5 years. Those with values between 170 mg/dL and 199 mg/dL should have a repeat test. If the average value of the two tests is less than 170 mg/dL, the total blood cholesterol level should be reassessed within 5 years. A lipoprotein analysis should be done if the average cholesterol value from the two tests is 170 mg/dL or higher or if the result of the initial test was 200 mg/dL or greater.

- Adolescents who have a parent or grandparent with coronary artery disease, peripheral vascular disease, cerebrovascular disease, or sudden cardiac death at age 55 years or younger should be screened with a fasting lipoprotein profile.

- Treatment options are based on the average of two assessments of low-density lipoprotein cholesterol. Values less than 110 mg/dL are acceptable; values between 110 mg/dL and 120 mg/dL are borderline, and the lipoprotein status should be reevaluated in 1 year. Adolescents with values of 130 mg/dL or greater will need further evaluation.

EATING DISORDERS

All adolescents should be screened annually for eating disorders and obesity by determining weight and stature, calculating a body mass index (BMI) (Fig. 3), and asking about body image and eating patterns. For many young women, significant weight loss or preoccupation with dieting should alert the obstetrician–gynecologist to the possibility of an eating disorder. Additionally, test results of vital signs may help to confirm the suspicion of eating disorders and identify patients needing emergency hospitalization. The following general guidelines should be used (see "Eating Disorders" chapter for more detailed information):

- Adolescents should be assessed for organic disease, anorexia nervosa, or bulimia nervosa if any of the following are found:

    —Amenorrhea or abnormal menses

    —Refusal to maintain body weight at or above a normal weight for age and height

Weight kg (lb)	Stature m (in)																										
	1.24 (49)	1.27 (50)	1.30 (51)	1.32 (52)	1.35 (53)	1.37 (54)	1.40 (55)	1.42 (56)	1.45 (57)	1.47 (58)	1.50 (59)	1.52 (60)	1.55 (61)	1.57 (62)	1.60 (63)	1.63 (64)	1.65 (65)	1.68 (66)	1.70 (67)	1.73 (68)	1.75 (69)	1.78 (70)	1.80 (71)	1.83 (72)	1.85 (73)	1.88 (74)	1.90 (75)	1.93 (76)
20 (45)	13	13	12	12	11	11	10	10	10	9	9	9	8															
23 (50)	15	14	13	13	12	12	12	11	11	10	10	10	9	9	9	9	8											
25 (55)	16	15	15	14	14	13	13	12	12	12	11	11	10	10	10	9	9	9										
27 (60)	18	17	16	16	15	15	14	13	13	13	12	12	11	11	11	10	10	10	9	9								
29 (65)	19	18	17	17	16	16	15	15	14	14	13	13	12	12	12	11	11	10	10	10	10							
32 (70)	21	20	19	18	17	17	16	16	15	15	14	14	13	13	12	12	12	11	11	11	10	10						
34 (75)	22	21	20	20	19	18	17	17	16	16	15	15	14	14	13	13	12	12	12	11	11	11	10					
36 (80)	24	22	21	21	20	19	19	18	17	17	16	16	15	15	14	14	13	13	13	12	12	11	11	11				
39 (85)	25	24	23	22	21	21	20	19	18	18	17	17	16	16	15	15	14	14	13	13	13	12	12	12	11			
41 (90)	27	25	24	23	22	22	21	20	19	19	18	18	17	17	16	15	15	14	14	14	13	13	13	12	12	12		
43 (95)	28	27	25	25	24	23	22	21	20	20	19	19	18	17	17	16	16	15	15	14	14	13	13	13	12	12		
45 (100)	29	28	27	26	25	24	23	22	22	21	20	20	19	18	18	17	17	16	16	15	15	14	14	14	13	13	13	12
48 (105)	31	30	28	27	26	25	24	24	23	22	21	21	20	19	19	18	17	17	16	16	15	15	14	14	13	13	13	13
50 (110)	32	31	30	29	27	27	25	25	24	23	22	22	21	20	19	19	18	17	17	16	16	15	15	15	14	14	13	
52 (115)	34	32	31	30	29	28	27	26	25	24	23	23	22	21	20	20	19	18	18	17	17	16	16	15	15	14	14	
54 (120)	35	34	32	31	30	29	28	27	26	25	24	24	23	22	21	20	20	19	19	18	18	17	17	16	16	15	15	15
57 (125)	37	35	34	33	31	30	29	28	27	26	25	25	24	23	22	21	21	20	20	19	19	18	17	17	17	16	16	15
59 (130)	38	37	35	34	32	31	30	29	28	27	26	26	25	24	23	22	22	21	20	20	19	19	18	18	17	17	16	16
61 (135)	40	38	36	35	34	33	31	30	29	28	27	27	25	25	24	23	22	22	21	20	20	19	19	18	18	17	17	16
64 (140)	41	39	38	36	35	34	32	31	30	29	28	27	26	26	25	24	23	22	22	21	21	20	20	19	19	18	18	17
66 (145)	43	41	39	38	36	35	34	33	31	30	29	28	27	27	26	25	24	23	23	22	21	21	20	20	19	19	18	18
68 (150)	44	42	40	39	37	36	35	34	32	31	30	29	28	28	27	26	25	24	24	23	22	21	21	20	20	19	19	18
70 (155)	46	44	42	40	39	37	36	35	33	33	31	30	29	29	27	26	26	25	24	23	23	22	22	21	21	20	19	19
73 (160)	47	45	43	42	40	39	37	36	35	34	32	31	30	29	28	27	27	26	25	24	24	23	22	22	21	21	20	19
77 (170)	50	48	46	44	42	41	39	38	37	36	34	33	32	31	30	29	28	27	27	26	25	24	24	23	23	22	21	21
79 (175)		49	47	46	44	42	40	39	38	37	35	34	33	32	31	30	29	28	27	27	26	25	24	24	23	22	22	21
82 (180)		51	48	47	45	44	42	40	39	38	36	35	34	33	32	31	30	29	28	27	27	26	25	24	24	23	23	22
84 (185)			50	48	46	45	43	42	40	39	37	36	35	34	33	32	31	30	29	28	27	26	26	25	25	24	23	23
86 (190)				49	47	46	44	43	41	40	39	37	36	35	34	32	32	31	30	29	28	27	27	26	25	24	24	23
88 (195)				51	49	47	45	44	42	41	39	38	37	36	35	33	32	31	31	30	29	28	27	26	26	25	25	24
91 (200)					50	48	46	45	43	42	40	39	38	37	35	34	33	32	31	30	30	29	28	27	27	26	25	24
93 (205)						50	47	46	44	43	41	40	39	38	36	35	34	33	32	31	30	29	29	28	27	26	26	25
95 (210)							49	47	45	44	42	41	40	39	37	36	35	34	33	32	31	30	29	28	28	27	26	26
98 (215)							50	48	46	45	43	42	41	40	38	37	36	35	34	33	32	31	30	29	28	28	27	26
100 (220)								49	47	46	44	43	42	40	39	38	37	35	35	33	33	31	31	30	29	28	28	27
102 (225)								51	49	47	45	44	42	41	40	38	37	36	35	34	33	32	31	30	30	29	28	27
104 (230)									50	48	46	45	43	42	41	39	38	37	36	35	34	33	32	31	30	30	29	28
107 (235)										49	47	46	44	43	42	40	39	38	37	36	35	34	33	32	31	30	30	29
109 (240)										50	48	47	45	44	43	41	40	39	38	36	36	34	34	33	32	31	30	29
111 (245)											49	48	46	45	43	42	41	39	38	37	36	35	34	33	32	31	31	30
113 (250)											50	49	47	46	44	43	42	40	39	38	37	36	35	34	33	32	31	30
116 (255)												50	48	47	45	44	42	41	40	39	38	37	36	35	34	33	32	31
118 (260)													49	48	46	44	43	42	41	39	39	37	36	35	34	33	33	32
120 (265)													50	49	47	45	44	43	42	40	39	38	37	36	35	34	33	32
122 (270)														50	48	46	45	43	42	41	40	39	38	37	36	35	34	33
125 (275)															49	47	46	44	43	42	41	39	38	37	36	35	35	33
127 (280)															50	48	47	45	44	42	41	40	39	38	37	36	35	34
129 (285)															50	49	47	46	45	43	42	41	40	39	38	37	36	35
132 (290)																50	48	47	46	44	43	42	41	39	38	37	36	35
134 (295)																	50	49	47	46	45	44	42	41	40	39	38	36
136 (300)																		50	48	47	45	44	43	42	41	40	39	37

Fig. 3. Body mass index for selected weight and stature. (Reprinted with permission from: Guidelines for Adolescent Preventive Services [GAPS] Implementation Training Workbook. 2nd ed. Chicago, Illinois: American Medical Association, 1996.)

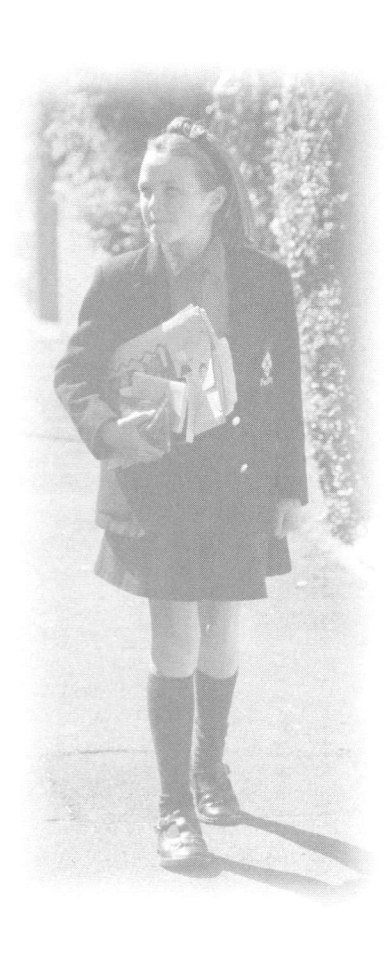

—Recurrent dieting when not overweight

—Use of self-induced emesis, laxatives, starvation, or diuretics to lose weight

—Distorted body image

—Body mass index below the 5th percentile

—Hypotension, bradycardia, cardiac arrhythmia, or hypothermia

- Adolescents with a BMI greater than or equal to the 95th percentile for age (Fig. 4) are overweight and should have an in-depth dietary and health assessment to determine psychosocial morbidity and risk for future cardiovascular disease.

- Adolescents with a BMI between the 85th and 94th percentile for age (Fig. 4) are at risk for becoming overweight. A dietary and health assessment to determine psychosocial morbidity and risk for future cardiovascular disease should be performed on these patients if:

—Their BMI has increased by two or more units during the previous 12 months

—There is a family history of premature heart disease, obesity, hypertension, or diabetes mellitus

—They express concern about their weight

—They have elevated blood pressure or cholesterol levels in serum

Tobacco

All adolescents should be asked annually about their use of tobacco products. Approximately 1 in 4 high-school seniors currently uses tobacco, and females are as likely as males to be smokers. Screening for tobacco use should include the following factors:

- Adolescents who smoke or use any tobacco products should be assessed further to determine their pattern of use.

- A cessation plan should be provided for adolescents who smoke or use any tobacco products. Appropriate nicotine therapy should be considered when there is strong evidence of nicotine dependence and a clear desire to quit tobacco use (12).

- Because of an adolescent's preoccupation with body image, all adolescents should be counseled on the effects of smoking and other tobacco products on their hair, skin, and breath.

- Counseling also should include long-term health consequences, including the possible impact on a female's reproductive potential.

Alcohol and Other Drugs

All adolescents should be asked annually about their use of alcohol and other drugs, including street drugs, over-the-counter and prescription drugs

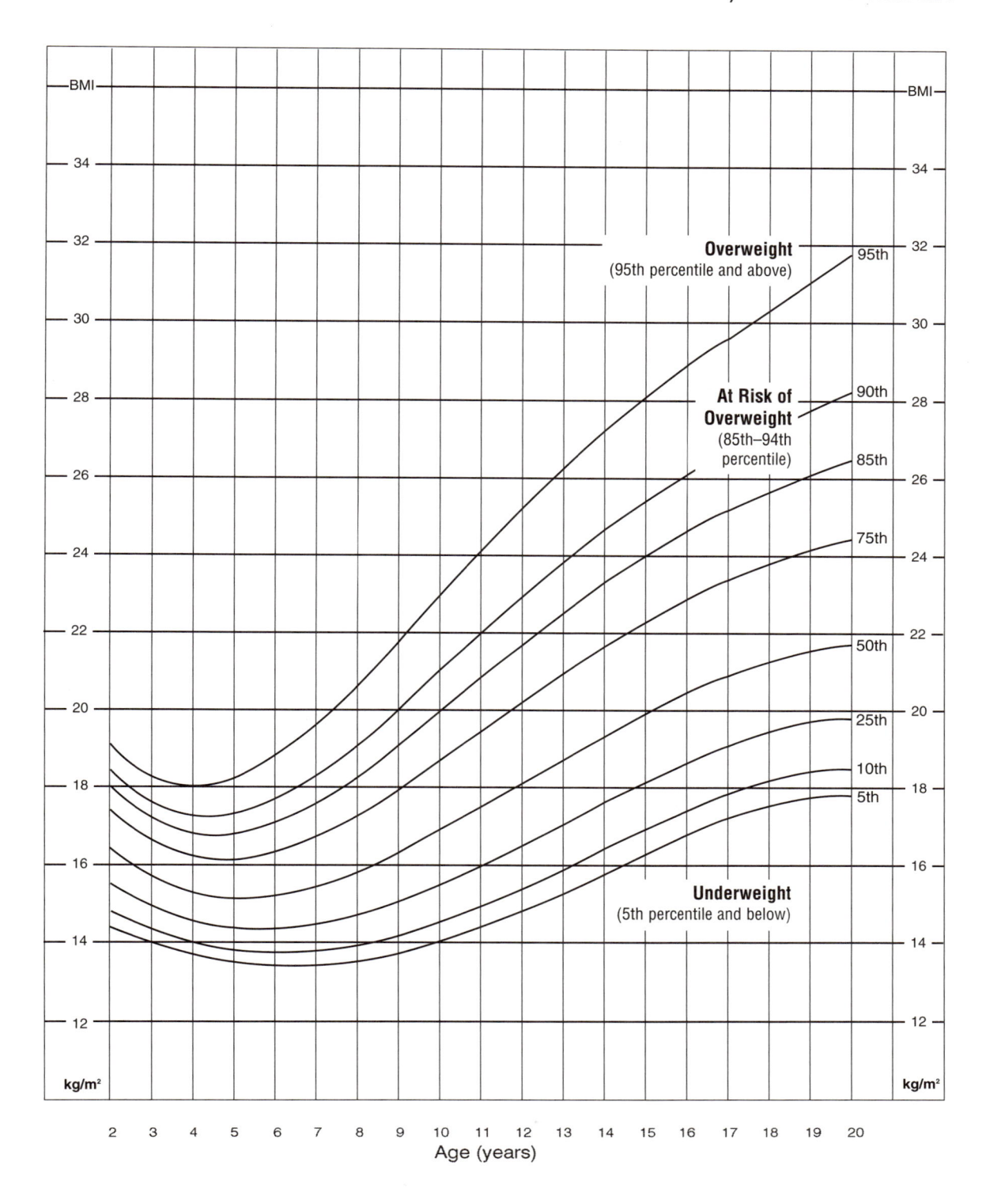

Fig. 4. Body mass index-for-age percentiles: Girls, 10 to 20 years. (Developed by the National Center for Health Statistics in collaboration with the National Center for Chronic Disease Prevention and Health Promotion [2000].)

for nonmedical purposes, and inhalants. Substance abuse occurs frequently in adolescence, is a major factor in injuries and deaths among adolescents, and contributes to motor vehicle accidents, homicide, and suicide. Screening for alcohol and drug use should include the following recommendations:

- Adolescents who report any use of alcohol or other drugs, or inappropriate use of medications during the past year should be assessed further regarding family history; circumstances surrounding use; amount and frequency of use; attitudes and motivation to use; use of other drugs; and the adequacy of physical, psychosocial, and school functioning.
- Adolescents whose substance use endangers their health should receive counseling and mental health treatment.
- Urine screening for drug use in adolescents without prior informed consent is not recommended and is illegal in many states.

SEXUAL ACTIVITY

All adolescents should be asked annually about their involvement in sexual behaviors that may result in unintended pregnancy and STDs, including HIV infection. High rates of sexual activity, coupled with inconsistent use of contraception, contribute to the United States having one of the highest adolescent pregnancy rates in the developed world. Currently, 1 out of every 10 adolescent females aged 15–19 years becomes pregnant annually (13).

Adolescents should be counseled that abstinence is the only health choice that assures protection from STDs and pregnancy. Sexually active patients must be educated about the safety and efficacy of current contraceptive options. The most effective protection against unintended pregnancy and STDs, other than abstinence, includes a combination of latex condoms and hormonal methods of birth control. Adolescents also should be counseled about emergency contraception pills. Although emergency contraception pills can prevent unintended pregnancies after episodes of unprotected sexual intercourse or method failure, they afford no protection against STDs. Pregnant adolescents whose pregnancies are unintended (either mistimed or unwanted) should be counseled about pregnancy options, including adoption, raising the baby, and termination. The practitioner must be knowledgeable about local support services and state laws regarding parental notification and consent for elective termination of pregnancy. If the adolescent continues with the pregnancy, the importance of prenatal care should be emphasized, and appropriate follow-up care should be arranged. For pregnant school-aged adolescents, the importance of completing high school should be stressed. Screening for sexual activity should include the following points:

- Sexually active adolescents should be asked about their sexual orientation, partner use of condoms, contraceptive methods, number of

current and previous sexual partners, exchange of sex for money or drugs, and history of prior pregnancy or STDs.
- Adolescents should be questioned about the age and the relationship with their partners to screen for possible sexual abuse.
- Adolescents at risk for pregnancy, STDs (including HIV), or sexual exploitation should be counseled on how to reduce their risk.

SEXUALLY TRANSMITTED DISEASES

Because most adolescent patients become sexually active before high school graduation, STDs are a major health issue for this population. Sexually transmitted diseases are the most common infectious diseases among adolescents and, as a group, they are at the greatest risk. Each year, nearly four million adolescents are infected with STDs, accounting for 25% of the 15 million new cases of STDs in the United States annually (14). As such, sexually active adolescents should be screened annually for STDs, including:

- Gonorrhea and chlamydia
- Syphilis if they have:
  — History of prior STDs
  — Multiple sexual partners
  — Exchanged sex for drugs or money
  — Used illicit drugs
  — Been admitted to jail or other detention facility
  — Lived in an endemic area
- Cervical neoplasia

HUMAN IMMUNODEFICIENCY VIRUS

All adolescents should be evaluated for their HIV risk status. Those found to be at risk should be offered HIV testing according to the following recommendations:

- Adolescents are at high risk if they have any of the following characteristics:
  — Multiple sexual partners
  — High-risk partner (eg, HIV positive, injectable drug user, bisexual, or has had more than one sexual partner)
  — Prior STDs
  — Exchange sex for drugs or money
  — Long-term residence or birth in an area with a high prevalence of HIV infection
  — History of blood transfusion before 1985
  — Use of intravenous drugs

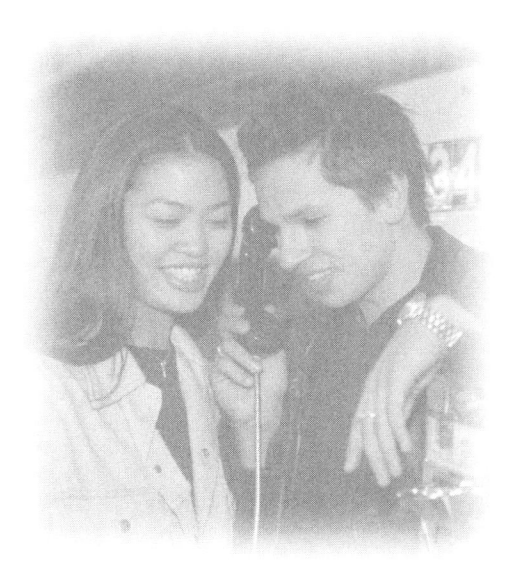

- Testing of nonpregnant adolescents should be performed only after informed consent is obtained, consistent with state legal requirements.
- Testing should be performed only in conjunction with both pretest and posttest counseling.
- The frequency of screening for HIV infection should be determined by risk factors.
- Universal HIV testing, with patient notification, should be a routine component of prenatal care for all pregnant adolescents. If the adolescent declines testing, this should be noted in the medical record (15).

DEPRESSION

All adolescents should be asked annually about behaviors or emotions that indicate recurrent or severe depression and a risk of suicide. Feelings of sadness should not be dismissed as mere moodiness in this patient population. Situational losses, relationship and school problems, parental loss, and parental conflicts may lead to depression. Recognition of depression and subsequent intervention can reduce suicidal behaviors in adolescent women. Recommendations for screening for depression are as follows (see "Preventing Adolescent Suicide" chapter for more information):

- Screening for depression or suicidal risk should be performed on adolescents who exhibit cumulative risk as determined by declining school grades, chronic sadness, family dysfunction, problems with sexual orientation, physical or sexual abuse, alcohol or other drug use, family history of suicide, previous suicide attempt, and suicidal plans.
- If suicidal risk is suspected, adolescents should be evaluated immediately and, based on their degree of risk, referred to a mental health professional or hospitalized.
- Nonsuicidal adolescents with symptoms of severe or recurrent depression should be assessed and, if necessary, referred to a mental health professional for treatment.

ABUSE

According to the Commonwealth Fund's Commission on Women's Health, 26% of adolescent girls in grades 9–12 report experiencing physical or sexual abuse, including date rape (9). Given this high incidence, all adolescents should be asked annually about a history of abuse, including emotional, physical, and sexual abuse. Following are screening recommendations:

- If abuse is suspected, adolescents should be questioned regarding the circumstances surrounding the abuse; assessed for physical, emotional, and psychosocial consequences; and screened for involvement in risky health behaviors.
- Health providers should be aware of local laws requiring breach of confidentiality and reporting of abuse to appropriate state officials.

- Adolescents who report emotional or psychosocial sequelae from abuse should be referred to a mental health professional for evaluation and treatment.

SCHOOL PERFORMANCE

All adolescents should be assessed annually for learning or school-related problems. Adolescents with a history of truancy, repeated absences, or poor or declining performance should be assessed or referred to other professionals to screen for the presence of conditions that could interfere with school success. These include learning disabilities, attention deficit hyperactivity disorder, medical problems, abuse, family dysfunction, mental disorder, and alcohol or other drug use. This assessment and the subsequent management should be coordinated with school personnel, the primary medical care provider (if different from the obstetrician–gynecologist), and the adolescent's parents or caregivers.

TUBERCULOSIS

Adolescents should be evaluated for their tuberculosis risk status. Adolescents should receive a tuberculin skin test if they:

- Have been exposed to active tuberculosis
- Have lived in a homeless shelter, been incarcerated, or lived in another long-term care facility
- Have lived in or come from an area with a high prevalence of tuberculosis, or lived with individuals known or suspected to have tuberculosis
- Are currently working in a health care setting
- Are HIV positive
- Are medically underserved or low-income status
- Have a history of alcoholism
- Have medical risk factors known to increase the risk of disease if infected

The frequency of testing depends on the individual adolescent's risk factors. Adolescents with positive tuberculin test results should be treated according to the treatment guidelines put forth jointly by the Centers for Disease Control and Prevention and the American Thoracic Society (16).

Immunization

National immunization policies have changed in response to the development of a vaccination against the hepatitis B virus and the resurgence of measles and rubella among adolescent and adult populations. All adolescents should receive prophylactic immunizations according to the guidelines established by the federally convened Advisory Committee on

26% of adolescent girls in grades 9–12 report experiencing physical or sexual abuse, including date rape...

Immunization Practices (17) (Fig. 5). Physicians should determine the numbers and types of previous vaccinations to assess the immunization needs of adolescents.

Ideally, all vaccinations should be administered at the scheduled 11–12-year visit. In many instances, however, it will be necessary for physicians to administer vaccines to those who have fallen behind the recommended schedule or who were older than 11–12 years when the recommendations were formulated. Before administering immunizations, physicians should ensure that, if required, the necessary parental consent has been obtained. Following are recommendations for determining what immunizations are needed:

- Adolescents should receive a bivalent tetanus–diphtheria vaccine booster at the 11–12-year visit if not previously vaccinated within 5 years. With the exception of the tetanus–diphtheria booster at ages 11–12 years, routine boosters should be administered every 10 years.
- Adolescents should receive a second dose of measles–mumps–rubella vaccine at ages 11–12 years, unless there is documentation of two vaccinations earlier during childhood. Measles–mumps–rubella vaccine should not be administered to pregnant adolescents.
- Hepatitis B immunization is administered in three parts and generally is provided to infants. Older children should be assessed and, if unvaccinated, should receive immunization at ages 11–12 years. The immunization status of older adolescents also should be assessed and the vaccine administered, if necessary (6).
- Hepatitis A vaccination should be given to adolescents who are traveling to or living in countries with high or intermediate endemicity of hepatitis A virus, live in communities with high endemic rates of hepatitis A virus, have chronic liver disease, or are injecting drug users.
- Varicella should be administered at the 11–12-year visit to all unvaccinated individuals or those lacking a reliable history of chickenpox. Susceptible individuals aged 13 years or older should receive two doses at least 1 month apart.

Summary

Although most adolescents enjoy good health, many of their behaviors put them at risk for negative health outcomes. Consequently, a fundamental change in the provision of health care services is required. Increasingly, services must be directed at primary and secondary prevention. As such, physicians should respond by making preventive services a greater component of their clinical practice. The approach outlined previously can help in this transition and can ensure that adolescents receive the services their health status demands.

Vaccine ▼ Age ▶	Birth	1 mo	2 mo	4 mo	6 mo	12 mo	15 mo	18 mo	24 mo	4–6 y	11–12 y	13–18 y
Hepatitis B[1]	Hep B No. 1	Only if mother HBsAg (-)									Hep B series	
			Hep B No. 2			Hep B No. 3						
Diphtheria, tetanus, pertussis[2]			DTaP	DTaP	DTaP		DTaP			DTaP	Td	
Haemophilus influenzae Type b[3]			Hib	Hib	Hib	Hib						
Inactivated polio[4]			IPV	IPV		IPV				IPV		
Measles–mumps–rubella[5]						MMR No. 1				MMR No. 2	MMR No. 2	
Varicella[6]						Varicella					Varicella	
Pneumococcal[7]			PCV	PCV	PCV	PCV				PCV	PPV	
Hepatitis A[8]										Hepatitis A series		
Influenza[9]						Influenza (yearly)						

Range of Recommended Ages | Catch-up Vaccination | Preadolescent Assessment

This schedule indicates the recommended ages for routine administration of currently licensed childhood vaccines, as of December 1, 2001, for children through age 18 years. Any dose not given at the recommended age should be given at any subsequent visit when indicated and feasible. ▇▇▇▇ Indicates age groups that warrant special effort to administer those vaccines not previously given. Additional vaccines may be licensed and recommended during the year. Licensed combination vaccines may be used whenever any components of the combination are indicated and the vaccine's other components are not contraindicated. Providers should consult the manufacturers' package inserts for detailed recommendations.

1. Hepatitis B vaccine (Hep B). All infants should receive the first dose of hepatitis B vaccine soon after birth and before hospital discharge; the first dose also may be given by age 2 months if the infant's mother is HBsAg-negative. Only monovalent hepatitis B vaccine can be used for the birth dose. Monovalent or combination vaccine containing Hep B may be used to complete the series; four doses of vaccine may be administered if combination vaccine is used. The second dose should be given at least 4 weeks after the first dose, except for Hib-containing vaccine, which cannot be administered before age 6 weeks. The third dose should be given at least 16 weeks after the first dose and at least 8 weeks after the second dose. The last dose in the vaccination series (third or fourth dose) should not be administered before age 6 months.

Infants born to HBsAg-positive mothers should receive hepatitis B vaccine and 0.5 mL hepatitis B immune globulin (HBIG) within 12 hours of birth at separate sites. The second dose is recommended at age 1–2 months and the vaccination series should be completed (third or fourth dose) at age 6 months.

Infants born to mothers whose HBsAg status is unknown should receive the first dose of the hepatitis B vaccine series within 12 hours of birth. Maternal blood should be drawn at the time of delivery to determine the mother's HBsAg status; if the HBsAg test is positive, the infant should receive HBIG as soon as possible (no later than age 1 week).

2. Diphtheria and tetanus toxoids and acellular pertussis vaccine (DTaP). The fourth dose of DTaP may be administered as early as age 12 months, provided 6 months have elapsed since the third dose and the child is unlikely to return at ages 15–18 months. Tetanus and diphtheria toxoids (Td) is recommended at ages 11–12 years if at least 5 years have elapsed since the last dose of tetanus and diphtheria toxoid-containing vaccine. Subsequent routine Td boosters are recommended every 10 years.

3. Haemophilus influenzae type b (Hib) conjugate vaccine. Three Hib conjugate vaccines are licensed for infant use. If PRP-OMP (Pedvax HIB® or ComVax® [Merck]) is administered at ages 2 and 4 months, a dose at age 6 months is not required. DTaP/Hib combination products should not be used for primary immunization in infants at age 2, 4, or 6 months, but can be used as boosters following any Hib vaccine.

4. Inactivated poliovirus vaccine (IPV). An all-IPV schedule is recommended for routine childhood poliovirus vaccination in the United States. All children should receive four doses of IPV at age 2 months, 4 months, 6–18 months, and 4–6 years.

5. Measles–mumps–rubella vaccine (MMR). The second dose of MMR is recommended routinely at ages 4–6 years but may be administered during any visit, provided at least 4 weeks have elapsed since the first dose and that both doses are administered beginning at or after age 12 months. Those who have not previously received the second dose should complete the schedule by the visit at 11–12 years.

6. Varicella vaccine. Varicella vaccine is recommended at any visit at or after age 12 months for susceptible children (ie, those who lack a reliable history of chickenpox). Susceptible persons aged 13 years or older should receive two doses, given at least 4 weeks apart.

7. Pneumococcal vaccine. The heptavalent pneumococcal conjugate vaccine (PCV) is recommended for all children aged 2–23 months and for certain children aged 24–59 months. Pneumococcal polysaccharide vaccine (PPV) is recommended in addition to PCV for certain high-risk groups. See MMWR 2000;49(RR-9);1–37.

8. Hepatitis A vaccine. Hepatitis A vaccine is recommended for use in selected states and regions, and for certain high-risk groups; consult your local public health authority. See MMWR 1999;48(RR-12);1–37.

9. Influenza vaccine. Influenza vaccine is recommended annually for children age 6 months or older with certain risk factors (including but not limited to asthma, cardiac disease, sickle cell disease, HIV, and diabetes; see MMWR 2001;50(RR-4);1–44), and can be administered to all others wishing to obtain immunity. Children aged 12 years or younger should receive vaccine in a dosage appropriate for their age (0.25 mL if aged 6–35 months or 0.5 mL if aged ≥3 years). Children aged 8 years or younger who are receiving influenza vaccine for the first time should receive two doses separated by at least 4 weeks.

Fig. 5. Recommended childhood immunization schedule—United States, 2002. (Centers for Disease Control and Prevention. Notice to readers: Recommended Childhood Immunization Schedule—United States, 2002. MMWR Morb Mortal Wkly Rep 2002;51:31–33.)

References

1. Grunbaum JA, Kann L, Kinchen SA, Williams B, Ross JG, Lowry R, et al. Youth risk behavior surveillance—United States, 2001. MMWR Surveill Summ 2002;51(SS-4):1–64.
2. Anderson RN. Deaths: leading causes for 2000. Nat Vital Stat Rep 2002;50(16):1–85.
3. Herman-Giddens ME, Slora EJ, Wasserman RC, Bourdony CJ, Bhapkar MV, Koch GG. Secondary sexual characteristics and menses in young girls seen in office practice: a study from the Pediatric Research in Office Settings Network. Pediatrics 1997;99:505–12.
4. Kaplowitz PB, Oberfield SE. Reexamination of the age limit for defining when puberty is precocious in girls in the United States: implications for evaluation and treatment. Drug and Therapeutics and Executive Committees of the Lawson Wilkins Pediatric Endocrine Society. Pediatrics 1999; 104:936–41.
5. Carnegie Council on Adolescent Development. Great transitions: preparing adolescents for a new century. Abridged version. New York: Carnegie Corporation of New York; 1996.
6. American College of Obstetricians and Gynecologists. Guidelines for women's health care. 2nd ed. Washington, DC: ACOG; 2002.
7. American Medical Association. Guidelines for adolescent preventative services (GAPS) recommendations monograph. Chicago (IL): AMA; 1997.
8. American College of Obstetricians and Gynecologists. Adolescent victims of sexual assault. ACOG Educational Bulletin 252. Washington, DC: ACOG; 1998.
9. The Commission on Women's Health. The Commonwealth Fund survey of the health of adolescent girls. New York: The Commonwealth Fund; 1997.
10. National High Blood Pressure Education Program. Update on the task force report (1987) on high blood pressure in children and adolescents: a working group report from the National High Blood Pressure Education Program. National Institutes of Health, National Heart, Lung, and Blood Institute. Bethesda (MD): National High Blood Pressure Education Program; 1996. NIH publication no. 96-3790.
11. National Cholesterol Education Program. Report of the Expert Panel on Blood Cholesterol in Children and Adolescents. National Institutes of Health, National Heart, Lung, and Blood Institute. Bethesda (MD): National Cholesterol Education Program; 1991. NIH publication no. 91-2732.
12. Fiore MC, Bailey WC, Cohen SJ, Dorfman SF, Goldstein MG, Gritz ER, et al. Smoking cessation. Clinical Practice Guideline No 18. Rockville (MD): U.S. Department of Health and Human Services, Public Health Service; 1996. AHCPR publication no. 96-0692.
13. Ventura SJ, Mosher WD, Curtin SC, Abma JC, Henshaw S. Trends in pregnancy rates for the United States, 1976–97: an update. Nat Vital Stat Rep 2001;49(4):1–9.
14. Cates W Jr. Estimates of the incidence and prevalence of sexually transmitted diseases in the United States. American Social Health Association Panel. Sex Transm Dis 1999;26(suppl 4):S2–7.
15. American Academy of Pediatrics, American College of Obstetricians and Gynecologists. Joint statement on human immunodeficiency virus screening. Elk Grove Village (IL): AAP; Washington, DC: ACOG; 1999.
16. Bass JB Jr, Farer LS, Hopewell PC, O'Brien R, Jacobs RF, Ruben F, et al. Treatment of tuberculosis and tuberculosis infection in adults and children. American Thoracic Society and the Centers for Disease Control and Prevention. Am J Respir Crit Care Med 1994;149:1359–74.

17. Recommended childhood immunization schedule—United States, 2002. MMWR Morb Mortal Wkly Rep 2002;51:31–3.

Resources

ACOG Resources

American College of Obstetricians and Gynecologists. Birth control—especially for teens. ACOG Patient Education Pamphlet AP112. Washington, DC: ACOG; 1997.

American College of Obstetricians and Gynecologists. Growing up—especially for teens. ACOG Patient Education Pamphlet AP041. Washington, DC: ACOG; 1997.

American College of Obstetricians and Gynecologists. Primary and preventive care: periodic assessments. ACOG Committee Opinion 246. Washington, DC: ACOG; 2000.

American College of Obstetricians and Gynecologists. Tool kit for teen care. Washington, DC: ACOG; 2003.

American College of Obstetricians and Gynecologists. You and your sexuality—especially for teens. ACOG Patient Education Pamphlet AP042. Washington, DC: ACOG; 1996.

American College of Obstetricians and Gynecologists. Your first ob-gyn visit—especially for teens. ACOG Patient Education Pamphlet AP150. Washington, DC: ACOG; 2001.

Other Resources

The following lists are for information purposes only. Referral to these sources and web sites does not imply the endorsement of ACOG. These lists are not meant to be comprehensive. The exclusion of a source or web site does not reflect the quality of that source or web site. Please note that web sites are subject to change without notice.

American Academy of Family Physicians
11400 Tomahawk Creek Parkway
Leawood, KS 66211-2672
Tel: (913) 906-6000
Web: www.aafp.org

American Academy of Pediatrics
141 Northwest Point Boulevard
Elk Grove Village, IL 60007-1098
Tel: (847) 228-5005
Fax: (847) 228-5097
Web: www.aap.org

American Medical Association
515 North State Street
Chicago, IL 60610
Tel: (312) 464-5000
Web: www.ama-assn.org

Society for Adolescent Medicine
1916 NW Copper Oaks Circle
Blue Springs, MO 64015
Tel: (816) 224-8010
Web: www.adolescenthealth.org

The Society of Obstetricians and Gynecologists of Canada
780 Echo Drive
Ottawa ON
Canada K15 5R7
Tel: (613) 730-4192; 800-561-2416
Fax: (613) 730-4314
Web: www.sexualityandu.ca

RESOURCES FOR YOUR PATIENTS

Center for Young Women's Health
Children's Hospital
333 Longwood Avenue, 5th floor
Boston, MA 02115
Tel: (617) 355-CYWH (2994)
Fax: (617) 232-3136
Web: www.youngwomenshealth.org

Go Ask Alice! (by Columbia University Health Education Program)
Lerner Hall
2920 Broadway, 7th Floor
MC 2608
New York, NY 10027
Tel: (212) 854-5453
Fax: (212) 854-8949
Web: www.goaskalice.columbia.edu

National Women's Health Information Center (by DHHS Office on Women's Health)
8550 Arlington Boulevard, Suite 300
Fairfax, VA 22031
Tel: 800-994-WOMAN
Web: www.4woman.org; www.4girls.gov

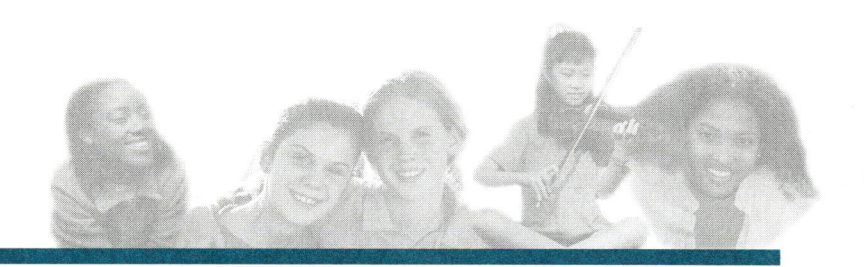

Confidentiality in Adolescent Health Care

KEY POINTS

- Concern about confidentiality is a major obstacle to the delivery of health care to adolescents.

- Physicians should address confidentiality issues with the adolescent patient to build a trusting relationship with her and to facilitate a candid discussion regarding her health and health-related behaviors.

- Physicians also should discuss confidentiality issues with the parent(s) or guardian(s) of the adolescent patient. Physicians should encourage their involvement in the patient's health and health care decisions and, when appropriate, facilitate communication between the two.

- Physicians should develop office procedures to maintain adolescent patients' rights for confidentiality. All office staff should be aware of these procedures.

- Physicians should be familiar with state and local statutes regarding the rights of minors to health care services and the federal and state laws that affect confidentiality.

- The right of a "mature minor" to obtain selected medical care, including services related to contraception, pregnancy, sexually transmitted diseases, and mental health, without parental consent has been established in most states.

- A minor's right to obtain an abortion without parental involvement is restricted in most states.

- Health care providers should work to ensure that confidential services for adolescents are not compromised by legal and economic constraints.

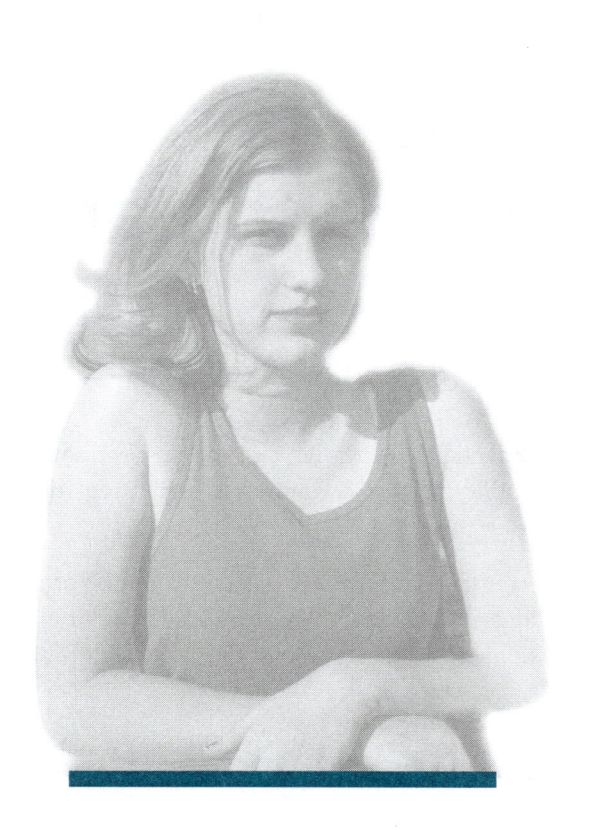

Adolescents are a relatively healthy subgroup of the U.S. population. Much of their behavior, however, puts them at substantial risk for poor health. Behaviorally related morbidities include alcohol and substance abuse; sexually transmitted diseases (STDs), including human immunodeficiency virus (HIV); pregnancy; depression; injury; violence; and suicide. Because these behaviors can jeopardize an adolescent's development, future opportunities, and even life, any barriers to needed health care services should be identified and removed.

Most adolescents underuse existing health care services. A major obstacle to the delivery of health care to adolescents is their concern about confidentiality. Confidentiality refers to the privileged and private nature of information shared during a health care encounter (1). Although ensuring confidentiality is relatively simple when providing services to adults, providing the same degree of confidentiality to adolescents can be less straightforward. The legal status of a minor and legal requirements for parental consent before the provision of medical services often encumber the physician–patient relationship.

Confidentiality also may be compromised by economic considerations because few adolescents have the financial resources to pay for medical services and, therefore, may need parental or adult help in arranging payment. Although a few states allow adolescents to qualify for Medicaid on the basis of their own incomes, the majority of states consider family income and assets when determining eligibility. To supply such information, adolescents may need to consult with family members. Explanation of Benefits forms issued by indemnity insurers, managed care organizations, and Medicaid are sent to parent policyholders, which also can compromise the confidentiality of information and, therefore, a minor's access to health care services.

To overcome barriers to confidentiality imposed by legal and economic constraints, physicians should discuss confidentiality with both the adolescent girl and, where appropriate, her parent(s) or guardian(s). Health care providers should be familiar with current state and local statutes on the rights of minors to consent to health care services, as well as those federal and state laws that affect confidentiality. It also is important to involve and inform office staff about those policies and procedures that facilitate and ensure confidentiality. Finally, physicians should work with the polit-

Confidentiality refers to the privileged and private nature of information shared during a health care encounter ...

ical process to eliminate laws unduly restrictive of confidential health services for adolescents.

Addressing Confidentiality

Parents should be counseled that it is appropriate for the maturing adolescent girl to assume increasing responsibility for her health and health care. Adolescence is a period of significant change and maturation, and learning to make appropriate health care decisions is a major developmental task. Physicians can assist in this process by providing an environment in which adolescents can candidly discuss their concerns. Adolescents are more likely to develop trusting relationships with their health care providers when the issue of confidentiality has been addressed. A confidential relationship, in turn, facilitates the open disclosure of health histories and risky behaviors. The health and behavioral issues of adolescent patients can then be addressed with nonjudgmental counseling and medical intervention.

Physicians should stress to parents that they share a common goal—the health and well-being of the minor patient. The mutual trust that follows from this common goal will enhance and support the adolescent–physician relationship. The involvement of a concerned adult can contribute to the health and success of an adolescent. Providers should encourage and, when appropriate, facilitate communication between a minor and her parent(s) (2).

Parents and adolescents should be informed, both separately and together, that they each have a private and privileged relationship with the provider. Additionally, they should be informed of any restrictions on the confidential nature of that relationship. For instance, the physician should explain that if the patient discloses any risk of bodily harm to herself or others (3), confidentiality will be breached. Furthermore, state laws may mandate the reporting of physical or sexual abuse of minors.

Legal Issues

Because the legal status of minors differs from that of adults, physicians who treat minors should be aware of laws that affect the provision of services. The following information is an introduction to the laws that address the medical treatment of minors. Providers of care to adolescents are encouraged to familiarize themselves with federal and state laws to determine which services mandate confidentiality. When necessary, they should seek appropriate legal advice.

All states require consent for the medical treatment of a minor from an individual legally entitled to authorize such care. Although this usually will be a parent, other guardians, such as foster parents, juvenile courts, social workers, and probation officers, may provide the necessary consent in certain instances.

There are, however, exceptions to this requirement for consent. Generally, where such exceptions apply, minors have the right to prevent physicians from disclosing information about the care they receive. First, in an emergency situation, when immediate treatment is necessary to safeguard the life or health of a minor, parental consent is assumed (4). Second, "emancipated minors" generally are held to be capable of consenting to medical treatment (4). Such minors may include those who are married, those who are members of the armed forces, those who live apart from their parents and are financially self-supporting, and those who are themselves the parent of a child. Third, all states and the District of Columbia have statutes allowing minors to consent to at least some specific health care services. These services may include contraceptive services, prenatal care and delivery services, STD services, HIV testing and treatment, treatment of drug and alcohol abuse, and mental health treatment (4). These laws may specify the age at which minors can begin to consent to such care.

In addition, courts increasingly recognize the growing independence of adolescents and the seriousness of their health care needs. Through case law, the right of a "mature minor" to consent to some forms of medical care without prior parental consent has been established. A mature minor is defined as an adolescent younger than the age of majority who, although living at home as a dependent, demonstrates the cognitive maturity to give informed consent (1). The age of majority has been set at 18 years in most states. The ability to consent will be influenced by the minor's developmental maturity, prior experience with illness, the gravity of the current illness, and the risks of proposed therapy (1). Although the mature-minor doctrine has been written into law in only a few states, during the past several decades there have been no reported decisions holding a physician liable solely for failing to obtain parental consent when nonnegligent care was provided to a mature minor (typically at least age 15 years) who had given informed consent (5). When dealing with high-risk health concerns, such as contraception, pregnancy, STDs, and mental health, most states have concluded that the need for confidential services outweighs parental rights of notification. When deciding whether or not to accept a mature minor as a patient, individual providers should evaluate their personal views. If a provider's views on confidentiality restrict the provision of services to a minor, the patient should be referred to another health care provider.

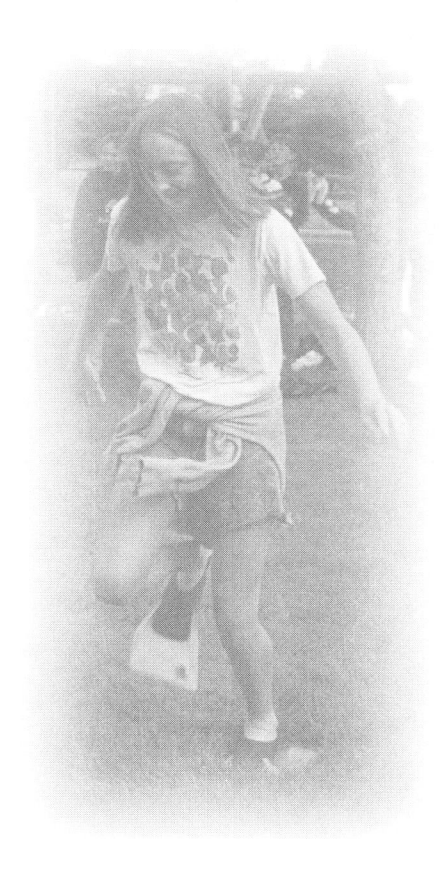

A minor's right to obtain an abortion without parental consent or notification is one area in which the rights of a minor have been statutorily restricted. As of this printing, 31 states have adopted either mandatory parental consent or mandatory parental notification laws. An additional 12 states have parental involvement laws that are blocked from going into effect. In all but one of the states where parental consent or notification is required for the termination of a minor's pregnancy, a confidential alternative to parental involvement is provided. This takes place typically in the form of a judicial bypass, which allows minors to seek consent from the court in lieu of a parent or guardian (6). The U.S. Supreme Court has ruled that if a minor chooses this option, the judge must consent to the procedure if he or she has determined the adolescent to be a "mature minor, or if termination of the pregnancy is in the minor's best interest" (7).

A Model Office Visit

Physicians should develop office procedures that safeguard their adolescent patients' rights. Furthermore, every member of the office staff must be aware of these procedures and their role in preserving confidentiality. Outlined in Table 1 and described as follows is an initial office visit process that works well when an adolescent girl is accompanied by her parent(s) or guardian(s):

1. The physician initially sees the parent and adolescent patient together to explain the structure of the visit. The reason for the visit and the patient's medical and family history are then reviewed. It is important to direct questions to, and maintain eye contact with, the adolescent patient during this discussion, deferring to the parent or guardian only when supplemental information or clarification is needed.

    The issue of confidentiality also should be discussed. Physicians should inform both the adolescent and her parent of the scope of the minor's authority to consent to medical care; physicians also should reassure them that family communication is encouraged and facilitated, and that no attempt is being made to undermine good parent–child relationships.

Table 1. An Adolescent Office Visit That Supports Confidentiality

In Consultation With	The Physician Should
Patient and parent(s) or guardian(s)	Outline structure of visit Obtain general medical and family history Discuss confidentiality
Patient	Obtain health history, including risk-taking behaviors Address patient concerns Provide health guidance Address billing issues
Parent	Address parental concerns Provide guidance about adolescent development
Patient*	Perform physical examination, as indicated
Patient	Summarize findings and recommendations Determine parental involvement Determine method of notification of laboratory results
Patient and parent(s) or guardian(s)	Summarize findings and recommendations, as appropriate Address billing issues

*Parent may be present, at patient's discretion

An adjunct to this discussion may be a simple written agreement (see Box 2). Such a document recognizes the adolescent's emerging autonomy and at the same time promotes communication between the parent(s) and child. It must be stressed that the agreement is not legally binding. It does, however, acknowledge the importance of confidentiality and outline the expectations of the new adolescent patient–parent–physician relationship. Parents also may be reminded that medical protocols may require pregnancy testing and screens for STDs when the adolescent has gynecologic concerns or complaints.

2. The parent(s) or guardian(s) should then be excused from the room. This allows for a confidential discussion between the physician and the patient about her health-related behaviors and concerns. The discussion about sexuality, substance abuse, alcohol, smoking, eating disorders, violence, depression, relationships, and school performance can be facilitated by adopting an open, relaxed, and nonjudgmental attitude. At this point it is important to distinguish between judging the behavior and judging the individual. Although certain behaviors can clearly be judged as negative or inappropriate, the adolescent patient should not be judged as "bad."

   Disclosures made during the discussion will determine the need for a physical examination. If a physical examination is necessary, the patient should be provided with a description of this process and asked if she would like her parent or another individual present.

3. While the patient prepares for the examination, a confidential meeting with the parent(s) or guardian(s) often proves beneficial. Parents may express specific concerns regarding their daughter's health, and physicians can provide them with a brief overview of adolescent development. Such a meeting often helps to relieve any anxiety parents feel in their new "passive" role. Physicians should reassure parents that they will encourage the adolescent to include her parents in important health decisions.

4. On completion of the physical examination, consultation with the patient should address physical findings and diagnosis and treatment options, if needed. Once a mutually agreed-on treatment plan is established, the adolescent is encouraged to include her parent in treatment planning. Depending on the adolescent's level of maturity, the nature of the medical problem, the physician's medical judgment, and legal constraints, parental involvement may be more or less strongly advised and facilitated. A method for reporting confidential laboratory results to the adolescent should be established at this time. If the adolescent agrees to parental input, and a conflict in treatment planning develops once the parents are involved, the physician often will have to take the role of arbitrator. Such a conflict may be resolved by determining if the adolescent has the legal right to consent to the services in question.

Box 2. Confidential Agreement

Parent

I, _____ (parent or guardian), allow

_____ (patient), to enter a confidential patient–physician relationship. I understand that she can make independent health care decisions, but that my input and involvement will be encouraged.

_____ (patient) has permission to schedule appointments and receive confidential reports from this office. I further understand that various laboratory tests may be necessary in medical protocols and accept responsibility for physician charges and laboratory fees.

_____
Parent or Guardian

_____
Physician

Patient

I, _____ (patient), am entering a confidential physician–patient relationship with

_____ (physician). I will make an effort to communicate with my parent(s) or guardian(s) about issues concerning my health. I accept the personal responsibility of being honest and will follow the health care recommendations my physician and I establish.

_____
Patient

_____
Physician

5. At the conclusion of the consultation with the patient, the patient, her parent, and the physician should meet again. During this meeting, findings and recommendations are discussed, if appropriate. Any remaining concerns also can be addressed.

6. Finally, a claim for payment is filed. Maintaining confidentiality for a minor patient often is a problem when billing for office visits and laboratory work for services such as pregnancy and STD testing. Insurance companies and health maintenance organizations may not reimburse for laboratory services described as "indicated routine screening" and may insist that parents receive an itemized bill listing the specific tests. The disclaimer that "these tests are necessary in medical protocols" may be sufficient to satisfy the concerns of some parents. To ensure confidentiality, however, some adolescents may choose to pay for these tests themselves. Some practitioners offer a reduced rate for these tests or refer patients to agencies that charge on a sliding scale according to income. If the service is covered by an insurer with whom the physician has a contract, allowing the patient to pay out-of-pocket could violate the terms of the contract because she is being denied a covered benefit. Office personnel should be cognizant of the issues of confidentiality with billing, reviewing claims with parents, and reporting laboratory results.

Patient preferences or special circumstances (eg, reading level, learning disabilities) may necessitate a modification of the initial office visit process, and physicians should allow additional time for separate patient and parent interviews. Although this process may take more time than an adult patient visit, in the long run it should result in fewer telephone calls from parents who do not fully understand their changing role in their adolescent daughter's health care or the nature of confidential services for minors.

Conclusion

Confidential health services promote the health and well-being of all adolescents. Legal requirements and economic constraints, however, impose significant barriers to confidential health services for adolescents. Both minors and providers consistently identify concerns about the lack of confidentiality as major obstacles to minors obtaining needed health care. Overcoming the obstacles imposed by such constraints is not difficult. Providers should broach discussions of confidentiality with minor patients and their parents or guardians, familiarize themselves with current state and local statutes affecting confidentiality, and develop office procedures aimed at maintaining confidentiality. Family communication is the desired goal, and health care providers are able to assist in this effort. Confidential care does not preclude working toward this goal. By showing concern both for a parent's desire to be involved in a daughter's health care decisions and for the minor's growing need for autonomy, physicians can aid in a minor's healthy transition from childhood to adulthood.

References

1. Confidential health services for adolescents. JAMA 1993;269:1420–4.
2. Mccabe MA, Rushton CH, Glover J, Murray MG, Leikin S. Implications of the Patient Self-Determination Act: guidelines for involving adolescents in medical decision making. J Adolesc Health 1996;19:319–24.
3. Gans JE. Policy compendium on confidential health services for adolescents. Chicago (IL): American Medical Association; 1993.
4. Boonstra H, Nash E. Minors and the right to consent to health care. Guttmacher Rep Public Policy 2000;3(4):4–8.
5. English A, Matthews M, Extavour K, Palamountain C, Yang J. State minor consent statutes: a summary. Cincinnati (OH): Center for Continuing Education in Adolescent Health; 1995.
6. The adolescent's right to confidential care when considering abortion. American Academy of Pediatrics. Committee on Adolescence. Pediatrics 1996;97:746–51.
7. Alan Guttmacher Institute. State policies in brief. Parental involvement in minors' abortions. New York: AGI; 2002. Available at: http://www.agi-usa.org/pubs/spib_PIMA.pdf. Retrieved October 10, 2002.

Resources

American College of Obstetricians and Gynecologists. Tool kit for teen care. Washington, DC: ACOG; 2003.

American College of Obstetricians and Gynecologists. Your first ob-gyn visit—especially for teens. ACOG Patient Education Pamphlet AP150. Washington, DC: ACOG; 2001.

OTHER RESOURCES

The following lists are for information purposes only. Referral to these sources and web sites does not imply the endorsement of ACOG. These lists are not meant to be comprehensive. The exclusion of a source or web site does not reflect the quality of that source or web site. Please note that web sites are subject to change without notice.

Alan Guttmacher Institute
120 Wall Street, 21st Floor
New York, NY 10005
Tel: (212) 248-1111
Fax: (212) 248-1952
Web: www.agi-usa.org/pubs/spib.html

American Academy of Family Physicians
11400 Tomahawk Creek Parkway
Leawood, KS 66211-2672
Tel: (913) 906-6000
Web: www.aafp.org

American Academy of Pediatrics
141 Northwest Point Boulevard
Elk Grove Village, IL 60007-1098
Tel: (847) 228-5005
Fax: (847) 228-5097
Web: www.aap.org

American Medical Association
515 North State Street
Chicago, IL 60610
Tel: (312) 464-5000
Web: www.ama.assn.org

Center for Adolescent Health and the Law
211 North Columbia Street
Chapel Hill, NC 27514
Tel: (919) 968-8870
Fax: (919) 968-8854
Web: www.adolescenthealthlaw.org

Society for Adolescent Medicine
1916 NW Copper Oaks Circle
Blue Springs, MO 64015
Tel: (816) 224-8010
Web: www.adolescenthealth.org

RESOURCES FOR YOUR PATIENTS

Go Ask Alice! (by Columbia University Health Education Program)
Lerner Hall
2920 Broadway, 7th Floor
MC 2608
New York, NY 10027
Tel: (212) 854-5453
Fax: (212) 854-8949
Web: www.goaskalice.columbia.edu

National Women's Health Information Center (by DHHS Office on Women's Health)
8550 Arlington Boulevard, Suite 300
Fairfax, VA 22031
Tel: 800-994-WOMAN
Web: www.4woman.org

Teenwire (by Planned Parenthood Federation of America)
810 Seventh Avenue
New York, NY 10019
Tel: (212) 541-7800
Fax: (212) 245-1845
Web: www.teenwire.com

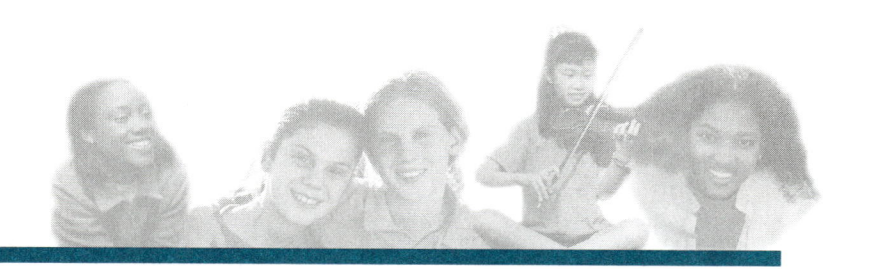

Oral Contraceptives for Adolescents: Benefits and Safety

Key points

➢ Oral contraceptives (OCs) are the most popular method of contraception among female adolescents. They are highly effective at preventing pregnancy when used correctly and consistently, but incorrect and inconsistent use of OCs is a substantial problem among adolescents.

➢ The initial visit for oral contraceptives does not have to include a pelvic examination if the patient requests that it be deferred. Adolescents need special attention at every visit for contraceptive services, including comprehensive counseling about sexuality, sexually transmitted disease prevention, and emergency contraception.

➢ Adolescents may be deterred from using OCs because of costs and concerns about confidentiality. Physicians should be familiar with the current state and local statutes regarding minors' rights on health care services and confidentiality.

➢ Oral contraceptives have a beneficial effect on many conditions common to adolescents, such as dysmenorrhea, benign breast disease, functional ovarian cysts, iron deficiency anemia, acne, and menstrual irregularity. Oral contraceptives also reduce the risk of ovarian and endometrial cancers, pelvic inflammatory disease, ectopic pregnancy, and toxic shock syndrome.

➢ Conditions contraindicating use of combination OCs are rare in adolescents.

➢ Adolescents may hesitate to use OCs or discontinue their use because of concerns about their complications and side effects. Physicians should address these concerns by proper counseling. Common sources of concerns include blood clots; cardiovascular disease; ovarian, breast, and cervical cancers; impaired fertility; stunted growth; weight gain; and menstrual irregularity.

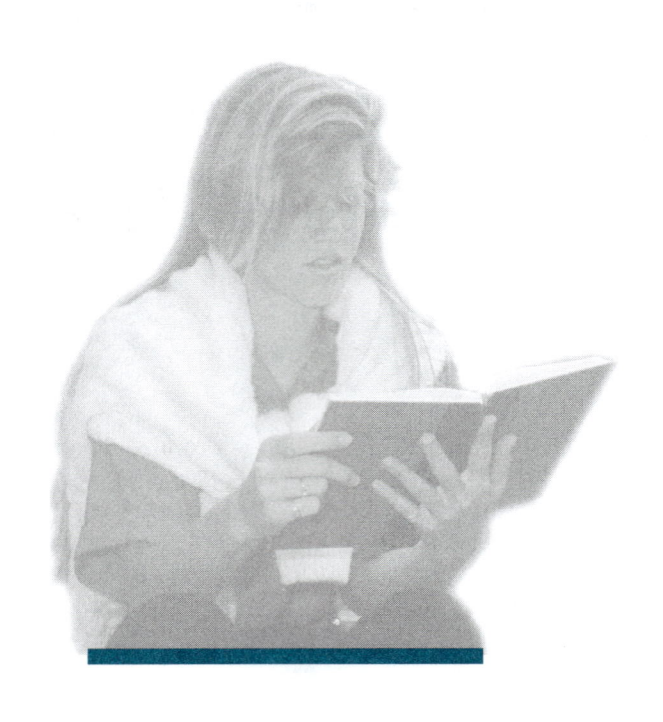

Correct and consistent use of all forms of contraception is an integral part of the prevention of adolescent pregnancy. The percentage of women using any method of birth control at first intercourse increased from 50% among those beginning coitus before 1980 to 76% for those beginning coitus in the 1990s (1). Oral contraceptives (OCs) are the most popular method of contraception among female adolescents. In a 1995 survey, 44% of adolescents at risk for pregnancy chose OCs compared with 37% who chose condoms, 10% who chose injectable contraceptives, and 3% who chose contraceptive implants (2). However, only 40% of adolescents seek medical contraceptive services within the first year of sexual activity (3).

Oral contraceptives are highly effective at preventing pregnancy when used consistently and correctly, with a reported failure rate of 0.1% (4). The failure rate of OCs for all women in the first year of use varies by age, income, and whether they are married, unmarried, or cohabiting. Low-income adolescents who cohabit have the highest OC failure rates (5). Adolescents are more likely to miss taking pills and may take OCs in an on-again, off-again fashion, depending on their patterns of sexual activity, which often includes serial monogamy (3, 6, 7). Only 40% of adolescents who use OCs took the pill every day and only 19% took it at the same time every day (3). The failure rate of OCs among adolescents is as high as 32% compared with 5% among all typical users (4, 5).

Special attention must be given to the adolescent during every visit for contraceptive services. Components of the initial visit should include comprehensive counseling and provision of information about human sexuality and the prevention of sexually transmitted diseases (STDs). The initial visit does not have to include a pelvic examination if the patient requests that it be deferred (8). Health care providers also should educate adolescents about the value of emergency oral contraception, explain how it is used, and consider providing an advance prescription (9). The information provided should be reinforced at subsequent visits.

Confidentiality concerns are a deterrent to the use of contraceptive services by adolescents and should be allayed during the heath care visit. As of this printing, 27 states and the District of Columbia have laws that explicitly give minors the authority to consent to contraceptive services (10). Pro-

...only 40% of adolescents seek medical contraceptive services within the first year of sexual activity.

viders should be familiar with current state and local statutes on the rights of minors to consent to health care services, as well as those laws that affect confidentiality. They also should encourage and, when appropriate, facilitate communication between a minor and her parent(s) (see "Confidentiality in Adolescent Health Care" chapter for more on confidentiality issues).

The costs associated with OCs also are a deterrent to adolescent use. To ensure confidentiality, adolescents who have insurance coverage through their parents may not want to use the benefit to obtain OCs. Others may be uninsured or have insurance that excludes coverage of OCs. In all of these cases, referral to a publicly funded clinic may be appropriate.

Benefits of Oral Contraceptives

In addition to preventing pregnancy, the health benefits of combination OCs for almost all healthy adolescents outweigh the minimal risks. There are a small number of individuals with specific medical conditions, such as a history of venous thromboembolism, for whom OCs containing estrogen are contraindicated. However, even for adolescents with medical conditions, such as diabetes mellitus, pregnancy may pose a much greater risk than OC use.

Combination OCs have a beneficial effect on a number of conditions that can affect an adolescent's quality of life, including dysmenorrhea, benign breast disease, functional ovarian cysts, iron deficiency anemia, acne, and menstrual irregularity. In the United States, adult women and adolescents remain misinformed about the health effects of OCs. In a 1998 survey, one half of the respondents were not aware of any OC benefits beyond preventing pregnancy (11).

Dysmenorrhea is one of the most frequent and debilitating conditions experienced by adolescents. Most women have moderate to complete relief within a few months after starting OC use (12). Adolescents who experience relief of dysmenorrhea are more likely to use OCs consistently and correctly (13). Studies have documented a significant reduction in the risk of benign breast disease among OC users (14). Similarly, numerous studies have documented a significant reduction in the frequency of functional ovarian cysts requiring surgery among users of high-dose monophasic OC pills with more than 35 µg of estrogen. These findings may be extended to users of newer OC pills with lower levels of hormones (15). Many adolescents have marginal iron stores and iron deficiency anemia is a common problem. Because menstrual flow and its duration are decreased by nearly 50% with the use of OCs, iron stores can increase significantly (12).

Acne improves significantly with most OC pill formulations. This is contrary to the common belief among adolescents that most OCs worsen acne. In particular, OCs containing third generation progestins may have an additional benefit for adolescents with acne. Based on the results of placebo-controlled randomized clinical trials of the triphasic norgestimate OC, the

U.S. Food and Drug Administration recently added treatment of acne to the labeling for this formulation (16).

Chronic anovulation, which may have its onset in the adolescent years, can be treated with OCs. Oral contraceptives not only induce regular cyclic menses, but also suppress the hormone imbalance that occurs with chronic anovulation. This has a positive effect on the lipoprotein profile, thereby theoretically decreasing the long-term risk of cardiovascular disease. Oral contraceptive use also interrupts the steady state effect of estrogen on the endometrium associated with anovulation, preventing dysfunctional uterine bleeding and endometrial hyperplasia (17).

Oral contraceptive use helps reduce the risk of life-threatening conditions, such as ovarian and endometrial cancers, pelvic inflammatory disease (PID), ectopic pregnancy, and toxic shock syndrome. Endometrial and ovarian cancers are rare among adolescents, but if OCs are taken for more than 1 year the protective effects last for at least 19 years after the discontinuation of use (18). Adolescents have the highest rate of hospitalization for PID in the United States. Oral contraceptives reduce the risk of developing PID by altering the cervical mucus (4, 19). Other mechanisms for this risk reduction may include altering the endometrial lining and decreasing the ascent of bacteria into the upper genital tract (19). Epidemiologic studies (although not specific to adolescents) also indicate that the risk of toxic shock syndrome is reduced by approximately 50% in OC users (20). Use of OCs also may improve bone mineral density in women who are hypoestrogenic because of eating disorders or extreme exercise, although concurrent psychologic management is essential (21).

Potential Deterrents to the Use of Oral Contraceptives

Fear of complications or side effects is a major deterrent to the use of OCs by adolescents, and many may not start taking OCs once they have been prescribed. Common fears may include blood clots, cancer, impaired fertility, absence of withdrawal bleeding, and stunted growth (22). Most of these fears are unfounded and must be addressed by proper counseling (see Box 3).

THROMBOEMBOLISM

Epidemiologic studies have shown an association between combination OC use by women of all ages and an approximate fourfold increased relative risk of venous thrombosis and embolism compared with nonusers (23). The increased risk of thromboembolism noted in women currently using OCs appears to be related to the estrogenic component. Although low-dose OCs carry less risk of thromboembolism than the higher dose preparations used in the past, increased risk remains. However, venous thromboembolism occurs considerably less frequently with the use of modern combination OCs than during pregnancy. The overall risk of death from thromboem-

> **Box 3. Common Concerns of Adolescents**
>
> Following are some of the common concerns of adolescents and an appropriate response to be given by the physician:
>
> - **I'm going to get fat if I go on the pill**—Some women gain weight, some women lose weight. With the pills we can prescribe now, weight gain isn't as much of a problem as it used to be. If it becomes a problem for you, we can try a different pill. Don't stop taking the pill, though. Call me and we can talk about our options, and remember you'll gain a lot more weight if you get pregnant.
>
> - **Pills are dangerous**—For most adolescents, it is very safe to take the pill. This is true even if you smoke, which I hope you don't. In fact, taking the pill lowers your risk of some cancers and many other health problems. Plus, it is less dangerous for you to take the pill than it is for you to be pregnant and have a child.
>
> - **My friend who is on the pill says she bleeds when she isn't supposed to**—The pill can cause what is called "breakthrough bleeding." Most breakthrough bleeding is caused by missed pills, but sometimes it happens in the first few months after you start taking the pill. It is not harmful to your health and usually stops after a few months if you are taking the pill correctly. If you are taking the pills every day at the same time and have this problem for more than a few months, come in and see me. Just don't stop taking the pill. We can always try another pill until we get one that is right for you.
>
> - **My friend who is on the pill doesn't get her period anymore**—Missing a period may happen, but it is even more likely that you will have a lighter flow, shorter periods, and less cramps. If you miss one period and have taken the pill correctly, you should keep taking the pill. If you have forgotten some pills and miss one period, call me, but keep taking the pill.
>
> - **The pill causes acne**—Actually, many pills help get rid of acne. If acne is a problem for you and the pills prescribed don't help it, call me and we'll try a different pill.
>
> - **You have to tell my parents I'm on the pill**—I understand that confidentiality is a big concern for you. We will keep this just between you and me, if that is what you want. I do want to encourage you, though, to talk with your parents about your decision to go on the pill.

bolic phenomena in adolescents is very low. There were too few cases in 1992 for the number to meet the standards of reliability (24). Thus, even with a small increase in relative risk, the absolute risk of death from thromboembolism among adolescents using the low-dose OC pills available today approaches zero (25). There also has been concern over the risk of thromboembolism associated with the use of third-generation progestogens. Although the differences in the rates of nonfatal venous thromboembolism are small and the use of these pills may be beneficial to some patients, the decision regarding their use should be left to the physician and the patient. It should be noted that the risk of thromboembolism in adolescents with factor V Leiden and other familial thrombophilic conditions is increased when they use OCs. However, routine screening of adolescents before initiating combination OCs is not currently recommended (26).

CARDIOVASCULAR DISEASE

The use of OCs in healthy nonsmoking adult women does not increase the risk of cerebrovascular disease (27) or myocardial infarction (28). These observations are reassuring regarding the safety of OC use in adolescent patients. Although adolescents, as well as all women, should be encouraged not to smoke, cigarette smoking does not contraindicate the use of combination OCs by adolescents as it does for women older than 35 years who smoke. This is because of the low risk of cardiovascular disease among adolescents.

Preexisting hypertension is considered to be a relative contraindication to OC use (29). The prevalence of hypertension in the United States is strongly related to age and to smoking, with the lowest rates in adolescents (30). The risk that OCs would precipitate hypertension is remote for adolescents (31).

CANCER

Women remain concerned about the risk of cancer associated with OC use despite compelling epidemiologic evidence that the use of OCs provides significant protection against endometrial and ovarian cancer (32). In a 1998 survey, 27% of the women surveyed indicated that OCs cause cancer (11). Many women, including adolescents, are concerned that OC use will increase their risk of breast cancer. A recent pooled analysis of data on breast cancer and OC use has clarified this relationship. This analysis combined data from 54 studies, including more than 53,000 breast cancer patients and more than 100,000 controls, with reassuring overall findings. No increased risk of breast cancer was associated with past (10 or more years since OC discontinuation) OC use, regardless of duration of use. The presence or absence of a family history of breast cancer did not affect these observations, nor did the use of OCs formulated with various types or doses of hormones (33).

The association of OC use and breast cancer in young women remains an ongoing controversy. A reanalysis of one large study revealed that women aged 20–34 years who had ever used OCs had a slightly increased risk of being diagnosed with breast cancer at a young age (34). In addition, a slightly elevated breast cancer risk has been noted with current or recent (within 10 years of stopping) OC use, but the background risk of breast cancer among adolescents and young women is extremely small (33, 35). This excess risk involves tumors less advanced clinically than tumors diagnosed in individuals who do not use OCs. Overall, these observations indicate that OC use does not cause breast cancer. The elevated risk associated with current or recent use is unexplained. Some speculate that this reflects surveillance bias; because OC users are more likely to have contact with the health care system, tumors are detected earlier.

CERVICAL NEOPLASIA

The unique epidemiology of cervical neoplasias, similar to that of an STD, makes assessing any association with OC use challenging. However, recent publication of studies that control for potential confounding factors, including STD risk factors and cytology screening, have clarified our understanding of this subject. Several recent case–control studies found that the risk of invasive cervical cancer with OC use was not significantly different than in nonusers (36–38). Likewise, recent well-controlled studies have found no association between OC use and cervical intraepithelial neoplasia (CIN) (38, 39). Most studies have found no association between OC use and genital human papillomavirus infection (40–43). Adenocarcinoma, which accounts for approximately 10% of cervical cancers, may have an epidemiology distinct from that of the more common squamous tumor. Two large and well-controlled studies found that OC use was associated with a significantly increased relative risk of cervical adenocarcinoma (37, 44); the absolute risk is extremely small. From 1992 to 1996, the age-specific rate was 1 in 350,000 females aged 15–19 years (35).

All adolescents at risk for cervical neoplasia (those who have had intercourse), including those who use OCs, should receive regular cytology screening. Adolescents with a history of CIN (including those who have had conization, cryotherapy, or laser or loop excision) as well as those being evaluated for CIN remain appropriate candidates for OCs.

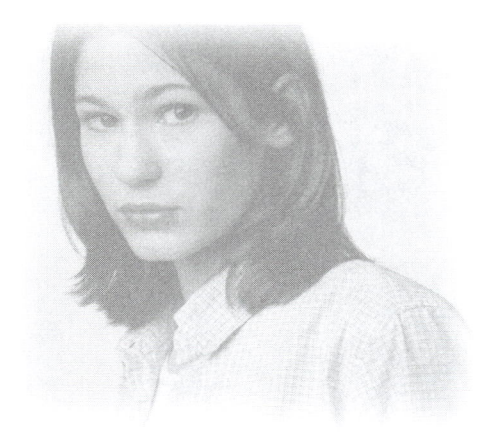

Amenorrhea and Delayed Fertility

Rather than causing oligomenorrhea or amenorrhea, OCs merely mask it by inducing cyclic withdrawal bleeding (29). The risk of amenorrhea after OC pill discontinuation is less than 1% and appears to be more common in women who had irregular menses before using OCs. Misunderstanding about the rapid resumption of ovulation has led to many unplanned pregnancies among adolescents who mistakenly believe that protection against pregnancy lasts several months after discontinuing OCs (45).

Effect on Height

Medical providers and parents may fear that OC use by adolescents will stunt physical growth. Oral contraceptives do not cause premature closure of the epiphyses or inhibit skeletal growth. By the time menarche occurs, endogenous estrogen production has already initiated epiphyseal closure, and this process cannot be altered by exogenous steroids (46). Therefore, use of OCs after menarche is appropriate.

Contraindications

Conditions contraindicating the use of combination OCs are rarely encountered in adolescents. Clinicians should be aware of contraindications listed in package labeling for OCs. In addition, progestin-only methods (including injections, implants, and progestin-only pills or mini-pills) may be more appropriate than combination OCs in adolescents with the rare conditions of refractory hypertension, severe hypertriglyceridemia, systemic lupus erythematosus associated with renal disease or antiphospholipid antibodies, and those with migraine headaches. Although progestin-only pills may be helpful in specific medical circumstances, they are prescribed infrequently, particularly for adolescents, because their efficacy is even more dependent on consistent and correct use than are combination OCs.

Causes of Discontinuation

Weight

Adolescents are extremely sensitive about their appearance, and weight gain related to OCs was a major worry for 85% of suburban adolescents in one study (47). Even the perception of weight gain as a side effect may result in discontinuation of OCs. Weight gain is infrequent with low-dose OCs. Placebo-controlled studies with high-dose OCs show similar rates of weight gain in the OC and placebo groups (48). In addition, a randomized, blinded clinical trial of a triphasic norgestimate–ethinyl estradiol OC found that the occurrence of weight gain was similar in the OC and placebo groups (49).

MENSTRUAL IRREGULARITIES

The side effects of breakthrough bleeding and failure to experience withdrawal bleeding can cause anxiety and are common reasons for OC discontinuation (47). Adolescents should be counseled that breakthrough bleeding is most common in the first months of use, is not medically harmful, frequently is caused by missed pills, and tends to resolve within a few cycles. Physicians should be aware that OCs formulated with 20 mg of estrogen are associated with substantially more breakthrough bleeding than OCs formulated with 30–35 mg of estrogen (50). Although lack of withdrawal bleeding can occur with consistent pill use, it should be investigated in adolescents to rule out pregnancy, given their high rates of missed pills. There is no substantive evidence that the use of any contraception during early pregnancy is associated with fetal anomalies. If a pregnancy occurs while OCs are being used, the method should be discontinued (9).

Irregular bleeding in adolescents using OCs can be caused by missed pills, incorrect use of the pill, cervicitis, endometritis, and neoplasia (51). Adolescents who experience irregular bleeding should be screened for pregnancy and STDs and counseled about consistent pill use.

OTHER SIDE EFFECTS

Other side effects of OC use, such as nausea, breast tenderness, and headache, may prompt an individual to discontinue usage. These side effects are rare with lower dose OCs. These symptoms often resolve spontaneously and can be managed with reassurance. If these side effects persist after 2–3 cycles, an alternative OC pill can be chosen.

Sexually Transmitted Diseases

Oral contraceptives are not intended to provide protection against STDs. Nearly 87% of girls and 80% of boys aged 15–17 years report considerable knowledge about STDs. However, these adolescents radically underestimate the incidence of STDs and possibly their risk of becoming infected (52). Sexually transmitted diseases affect four million adolescents annually (53). The common adolescent behavior of serial monogamy exposes each partner indirectly to infections of previous partners and emphasizes the need for education about STDs, including information about human immunodeficiency virus (HIV) infection and its prevention. There also are data suggesting that adolescent girls who use hormonal contraception, such as OCs, are less likely to use condoms (54). Dispensing condoms and demonstrating their correct use is important whenever OCs are prescribed (55).

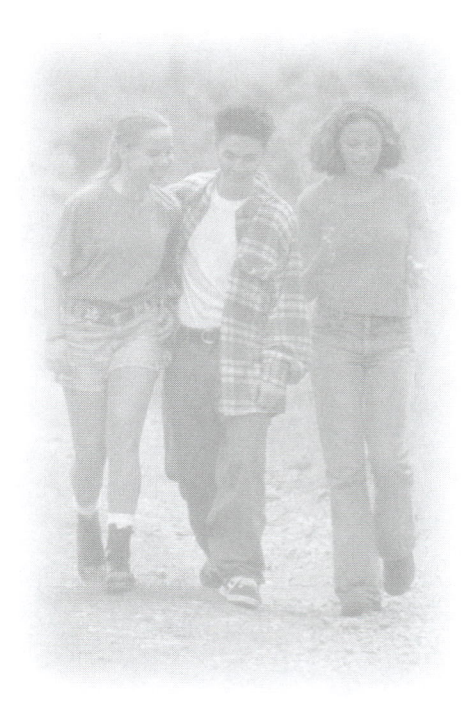

Encouraging Correct and Consistent Use of Oral Contraceptives

Oral contraceptives can be initiated on either the first day of menses or the first Sunday after menses begins. Oral contraceptives packaged with 28 pills facilitate consistent daily pill taking. Likewise, advising patients to associate pill taking with a daily ritual (eg, toothbrushing) may enhance compliance. Compliance is critical to ensure efficacy of OCs and is a particular problem for adolescents.

Patients should be told what to do when a pill is missed. If a woman misses one or two combination OC tablets, she should take one tablet as soon as possible. She should then continue to take one tablet twice daily until each of the missed tablets has been taken. If more than two consecutive tablets are missed, an additional form of contraception (eg, condoms and spermicide) is advised while they complete taking the current pack of pills. Because of the increased risk of accidental pregnancy, adolescents who consistently miss three or more combination OC tablets each cycle should be advised to consider other contraceptive choices that do not require daily compliance, such as injectable or implantable methods.

Postpartum Use

Pregnant adolescents should be counseled before delivery about the need for contraception postpartum. All options, including OCs, should be discussed. Progesterone-only pills or mini-pills do not appear to have adverse effects on lactation and may be useful in the postpartum months during lactation (56). Package labeling for norethindrone mini-pills has been updated. Patient instructions now state that this formulation can be started within 3 weeks postpartum in women who are partially nursing and at 6 weeks in those who are nursing exclusively (57). Mini-pills must be taken according to a rigorous daily schedule (17) and should be prescribed for adolescents with caution and counseling.

Summary

In the United States, adolescent pregnancy rates are higher than in nearly all other industrialized nations of the world despite comparable levels of sexual activity (3). Nearly one half (43%) of female high school students have had sexual intercourse (58). In the United States, approximately 870,000 pregnancies occurred in females aged 15–19 years in 1997 (59). Of these pregnancies, approximately 56% resulted in births, 29% in induced abortions, and 15% in spontaneous abortion or stillbirths (59).

Pregnancy rates among those adolescents who are sexually active have decreased while the use of contraceptives has increased (60). Oral contraceptives remain the most popular method of contraception among female adolescents. Sexually active adolescents should be advised to use condoms consistently with OCs to decrease their risk of STDs, including HIV infection. Adolescents who are not sexually active should be encouraged to remain abstinent.

For almost all adolescents, the benefits associated with the use of OCs for pregnancy prevention outweigh the medical risks. Adolescent compliance with OCs remains a substantial problem. Health care providers have the capacity to reduce this problem and help adolescents avoid the potentially disastrous outcome of an unintended pregnancy by educating them about the need for using OCs consistently, explaining the appropriate way to take OCs and respond to a missed pill, and allaying fears about side effects.

References

1. Abma JC, Chandra A, Mosher WD, Peterson LS, Piccinino LJ. Fertility, family planning, and women's health: new data from the 1995 National Survey of Family Growth. Vital Health Stat 23 1997;(19):1–114.
2. Piccinino LJ, Mosher WD. Trends in contraceptive use in the United States: 1982–1995. Fam Plann Perspect 1998;30:4–10, 46.
3. Alan Guttmacher Institute. Sex and America's teenagers. New York: AGI; 1994.
4. Hatcher RA, Trussell J, Stewart F, Cates W, Stewart GK, Guest F, et al. Contraceptive technology. 17th ed. New York: Ardent Media Inc; 1998.
5. Fu H, Darroch JE, Haas T, Ranjit N. Contraceptive failure rates: new estimates from the 1995 National Survey of Family Growth. Fam Plann Perspect 1999;31:56–63.
6. Oakley D, Sereika S, Bogue EL. Oral contraceptive pill use after an initial visit to a family planning clinic. Fam Plann Perspect 1991;23:150–4.
7. Hillard PJ. The patient's reaction to side effects of oral contraceptives. Am J Obstet Gynecol 1989;161:1412–5.
8. American College of Obstetricians and Gynecologists. Guidelines for women's health care. 2nd ed. Washington, DC: ACOG; 2002.
9. American College of Obstetricians and Gynecologists. Emergency oral contraception. ACOG Practice Bulletin 25. Washington, DC: ACOG; 2001.
10. Alan Guttmacher Institute. State policies in brief. Minors' access to contraceptive services. New York: AGI; 2002. Available at http://www.agi-usa.org/pubs/spib_MACS.pdf. Retrieved December 30, 2002.
11. Association of Professors of Gynecology and Obstetrics. Gallup survey finds health benefits are the best kept secret of the pill (press release). Washington, DC: APGO; October 6, 1998.
12. Larsson G, Milsom I, Lindstedt G, Rybo G. The influence of a low-dose combined oral contraceptive on menstrual blood loss and iron status. Contraception 1992;46:327–34.
13. Robinson JC, Plichta S, Weisman CS, Nathanson CA, Ensminger M. Dysmenorrhea and use of oral contraceptives in adolescent women attending a family planning clinic. Am J Obstet Gynecol 1992;166:578–83.
14. Charreau I, Plu-Bureau G, Bachelot A, Contesso G, Guinebretiere JM, Le MG. Oral contraceptive use and risk of benign breast disease in a French case-control study of young women. Eur J Cancer Prev 1993;2:147–54.
15. Lanes SF, Birmann B, Walker AM, Singer S. Oral contraceptive type and functional ovarian cysts. Am J Obstet Gynecol 1992;166:956–61.

16. Redmond GP, Olson WH, Lippman JS, Kafrissen ME, Jones TM, Jorizzo JL. Norgestimate and ethinyl estradiol in the treatment of acne vulgaris: a randomized, placebo-controlled trial. Obstet Gynecol 1997;89:615–22.
17. Speroff L, Darney PD. A clinical guide for contraception. 3rd ed. Philadelphia (PA): Lippincott Williams and Wilkins; 2001.
18. Rosenberg L, Palmer JR, Zauber AG, Warshauer ME, Lewis JL Jr, Strom BL, et al. A case-control study of oral contraceptive use and invasive epithelial ovarian cancer. Am J Epidemiol 1994;139:654–61.
19. Panser LA, Phipps WR. Type of oral contraceptive in relation to acute, initial episodes of pelvic inflammatory disease. Contraception 1991;43:91–9.
20. Gray RH. Toxic shock syndrome and oral contraception [letter]. Am J Obstet Gynecol 1987;156:1038.
21. Hergenroeder AC, Smith EO, Shypailo R, Jones LA, Klish WJ, Ellis K. Bone mineral changes in young women with hypothalamic amenorrhea treated with oral contraceptives, medroxyprogesterone, or placebo over 12 months. Am J Obstet Gynecol 1997;176:1017–25.
22. Rosenberg M, Waugh MS. Causes and consequences of oral contraceptive noncompliance. Am J Obstet Gynecol 1999;180:276–9.
23. Carr BR, Ory H. Estrogen and progestin components of oral contraceptives: relationship to vascular disease. Contraception 1997;55:267–72.
24. National Center for Health Statistics. Vital Statistics of the United States, 1992. Vol II, Mortality, part A. Washington, DC: Public Health Service; 1996; DHHS Publication No. (PHS) 96-1101.
25. Porter JB, Jick H, Walker AM. Mortality among oral contraceptive users. Obstet Gynecol 1987;70:29–32.
26. Kaunitz AM. Oral contraceptive use and venous thromboembolism: translating epidemiologic data into clinical practice. ACOG Clin Rev 1999;4(4):1–2, 11–2.
27. Petitti DB, Sidney S, Bernstein A, Wolf S, Quesenberry C, Ziel HK. Stroke in users of low-dose oral contraceptives. N Engl J Med 1996;335:8–15.
28. Sidney S, Siscovick DS, Petitti DB, Schwartz SM, Quesenberry CP, Psaty BM, et al. Myocardial infarction and use of low-dose oral contraceptives: a pooled analysis of 2 US studies. Circulation 1998;98:1058–63.
29. Andrews WC. Principles of oral contraception. In: Corson SL, Derman RJ, Tyrer LB, eds. Fertility control. Boston: Little, Brown; 1985. p. 157–69.
30. Benson V, Marano MA. Current estimates from the National Health Interview Survey, 1995. Vital Health Stat 10 1998;199:1–428.
31. Petitti DB, Klatsky AL. Malignant hypertension in women aged 15 to 44 years and its relation to cigarette smoking and oral contraceptives. Am J Cardiol 1983;52:297–8.
32. Grimes DA, Economy KE. Primary prevention of gynecologic cancers. Am J Obstet Gynecol 1995;172:227–35.
33. Breast cancer and hormonal contraceptives: collaborative reanalysis of individual data on 53,297 women with breast cancer and 100,239 women without breast cancer from 54 epidemiological studies. Collaborative Group on Hormonal Factors in Breast Cancer. Lancet 1996;347:1713–27.
34. Wingo PA, Lee NC, Ory HW, Beral V, Peterson HB, Rhodes P. Age-specific differences in the relationship between oral contraceptive use and breast cancer. Obstet Gynecol 1991;78:161–70.
35. Reis LA, Eisner MP, Kosary CL, Hankey BF, Miller BA, Clegg L, et al, editors. SEER cancer statistics review, 1973–1999. Bethesda (MD): National Cancer Institute; 2002. Available at http://seer.cancer.gov/csr/1973-1999/. Retrieved October 16, 2002.
36. Parazzini F, la Vecchia C, Negri E, Maggi R. Oral contraceptive use and invasive cervical cancer. Int J Epidemiol 1990;19:259–63.

37. Brinton LA, Reeves WC, Brenes MM, Herrero R, de Britton RC, Gaitan E, et al. Oral contraceptive use and risk of invasive cervical cancer. Int J Epidemiol 1990;19:4–11.
38. Kjaer SK, Engholm G, Dahl C, Bock JE, Lynge E, Jensen OM. Case-control study of risk factors for cervical squamous-cell neoplasia in Denmark. III. Role of oral contraceptive use. Cancer Causes Control 1993;4:513–9.
39. Coker AL, McCann MF, Hulka BS, Walton LA. Oral contraceptive use and cervical intraepithelial neoplasia. J Clin Epidemiol 1992;45:1111–8.
40. Ley C, Bauer HM, Reingold A, Schiffman MH, Chambers JC, Tashiro CJ, et al. Determinants of genital human papillomavirus infection in young women. J Natl Cancer Inst 1991;83:997–1003.
41. Bauer HM, Hildesheim A, Schiffman MH, Glass AG, Rush BB, Scott DR, et al. Determinants of genital human papillomavirus infection in low-risk women in Portland, Oregon. Sex Transm Dis 1993;20:274–8.
42. Wheeler CM, Parmenter CA, Hunt WC, Becker TM, Greer CE, Hildesheim A, et al. Determinants of genital human papillomavirus infection among cytologically normal women attending the University of New Mexico student health center. Sex Transm Dis 1993;20:286–9.
43. Fairley CK, Chen S, Ugoni A, Tabrizi SN, Forbes A, Garland SM. Human papillomavirus infection and its relationship to recent and distant sexual partners. Obstet Gynecol 1994;84:755–9.
44. Ursin G, Peters RK, Henderson BE, d'Ablaing G III, Monroe KR, Pike MC. Oral contraceptive use and adenocarcinoma of cervix. Lancet 1994;344:1390–4.
45. Kisker EE. Teenagers talk about sex, pregnancy, and contraception. Fam Plann Perspect 1985;17:83–90.
46. Bolton GC. Adolescent contraception. Clin Obstet Gynecol 1981;24:977–86.
47. Emans SJ, Grace E, Woods ER, Smith DE, Klein K, Merola J. Adolescents' compliance with the use of oral contraceptives. JAMA 1987;257:3377–81.
48. Goldzieher JW, Moses LE, Averkin E, Scheel C, Taber BZ. A placebo-controlled double-blind crossover investigation of the side effects attributed to oral contraceptives. Fertil Steril 1971;22:609–23.
49. Lippman JS, Godwin A, Olson W. The tolerability of a triphasic norgestimate/EE-containing OC: results from a double-blind, placebo-controlled trial. Prim Care Update Ob Gyns 1998;5:173–4.
50. Sulak P, Lippman J, Siu C, Massaro J, Godwin A. Clinical comparison of triphasic norgestimate 35 micrograms ethinyl estradiol and monophasic norethindrone acetate 20 micrograms ethinyl estradiol. Cycle control, lipid effects, and user satisfaction. Contraception 1999;59:161–6.
51. Krettek JE, Arkin SI, Chaisilwattana P, Monif GR. Chlamydia trachomatis in patients who used oral contraceptives and had intermenstrual spotting. Obstet Gynecol 1993;81:728–31.
52. The Henry J. Kaiser Family Foundation. What teens know and don't (but should) about sexually transmitted diseases: a national survey of 15 to 17 year-olds. Menlo Park (CA): Kaiser Family Foundation; 1999. Available at http://www.kff.org/content/archive/1465/std_cp.pdf. Retrieved October 16, 2002.
53. American Social Health Association. Sexually transmitted diseases in America: how many cases and at what cost? Menlo Park (CA): Kaiser Family Foundation; 1998. Available at http://www.kff.org/content/archive/1445/std_rep.pdf. Retrieved October 16, 2002.
54. Roye CF. Condom use by Hispanic and African-American adolescent girls who use hormonal contraception. J Adolesc Health 1998;23:205–11.

55. Rosenfeld WD, Bassoon Swedler J. Role of hormonal contraceptives in prevention of pregnancy and sexually transmitted diseases. Adolesc Med 1992;3:207–22.
56. American Academy of Pediatrics, American College of Obstetricians and Gynecologists. Guidelines for perinatal care. 5th ed. Elk Grove Village (IL): AAP; Washington, DC: ACOG; 2002.
57. Kaunitz AM. Revisiting progestin-only OCs. Contemp Ob Gyn 1997;42(12): 91–2, 97–8, 101.
58. Grunbaum JA, Kann L, Kinchen SA, Williams B, Ross JG, Lowry R, et al. Youth risk behavior surveillance—United States, 2001. MMWR Surveill Summ 2002;51(4):1–62.
59. Ventura SJ, Mosher WD, Curtin SC, Abma JC, Henshaw S. Trends in pregnancy rates for the United States, 1979-97: an update. Natl Vital Stat Rep 2001;49(4):1–9.
60. Saul R. Teen pregnancy: progress meets politics. Guttmacher Rep Public Policy 1999;2(3):6–9.

Resources

ACOG Resources

American College of Obstetricians and Gynecologists. Anticoncepción. ACOG Patient Education Pamphlet SP005. Washington, DC: ACOG; 2000.

American College of Obstetricians and Gynecologists. Birth control. ACOG Patient Education Pamphlet AP005. Washington, DC: ACOG; 1999.

American College of Obstetricians and Gynecologists. Birth control—especially for teens. ACOG Patient Education Pamphlet AP112. Washington, DC: ACOG; 1997.

American College of Obstetricians and Gynecologists. Birth control pills. ACOG Patient Education Pamphlet AP021. Washington, DC: ACOG; 1999.

American College of Obstetricians and Gynecologists. Emergency contraception. ACOG Patient Education Pamphlet AP114. Washington, DC: ACOG; 2000.

American College of Obstetricians and Gynecologists. Emergency oral contraception. ACOG Practice Bulletin 25. Washington, DC: ACOG; 2001.

American College of Obstetricians and Gynecologists. Tool kit for teen care. Washington, DC: ACOG; 2003.

American College of Obstetricians and Gynecologists. The use of hormonal contraception in women with coexisting medical conditions. ACOG Practice Bulletin 18. Washington, DC: ACOG; 2000.

Other Resources

The following lists are for information purposes only. Referral to these sources and web sites does not imply the endorsement of ACOG. These lists are not meant to be comprehensive. The exclusion of a source or web site does not reflect the quality of that source or web site. Please note that web sites are subject to change without notice.

American Academy of Family Physicians
11400 Tomahawk Creek Parkway
Leawood, KS 66211-2672
Tel: (913) 906-6000
Web: www.aafp.org

American Academy of Pediatrics
141 Northwest Point Boulevard
Elk Grove Village, IL 60007-1098
Tel: (847) 228-5005
Fax: (847) 228-5097
Web: www.aap.org

American Medical Association
515 North State Street
Chicago, IL 60610
Tel: (312) 464-5000
Web: www.ama.assn.org

American Society for Emergency Contraception
PO Box 1496
Princeton, NJ 08542
Tel: (609) 258-2661
E-mail: AmSocEC@aol.com

Association of Reproductive Health Professionals
2401 Pennsylvania Avenue NW, Suite 350
Washington, DC 20037-1718
Tel: (202) 466-3825
Fax: (202) 466-3826
Web: www.arhp.org

The Emergency Contraception Website and Hotline (by Princeton University Office of Population Research and the Association of Reproductive Health Professionals)
Tel: 888-NOT-2-LATE
Web: www.not-2-late.com

National Family Planning and Reproductive Health Association
1627 K Street NW, 12th Floor
Washington, DC 20006
Tel: (202) 293-3114
Fax: (202) 293-1990
Web: www.nfprha.org

Planned Parenthood Federation of America
810 Seventh Avenue
New York, NY 10019
Tel: (212) 541-7800
Fax: (212) 245-1845
Web: www.plannedparenthood.org

Society for Adolescent Medicine
1916 NW Copper Oaks Circle
Blue Springs, MO 64015
Tel: (816) 224-8010
Web: www.adolescenthealth.org

The Society of Obstetricians and Gynecologists of Canada
780 Echo Drive
Ottawa ON
Canada K15 5R7
Tel: (613) 730-4192; 800-561-2416
Fax: (613) 730-4314
Web: www.sexualityandu.ca

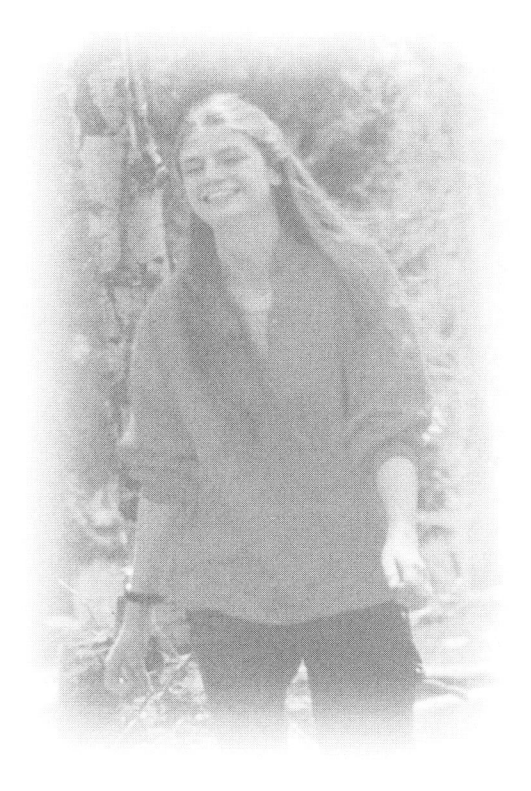

RESOURCES FOR YOUR PATIENTS

AWARE Foundation
1015 Chestnut Street, Suite 1225
Philadelphia, PA 19107-4302
Tel: (215) 955-9847
Web: www.awarefoundation.org

Center for Young Women's Health
Children's Hospital
333 Longwood Avenue, 5th floor
Boston, MA 02115
Tel: (617) 355-CYWH (2994)
Fax: (617) 232-3136
Web: www.youngwomenshealth.org

The Emergency Contraception Website and Hotline (by Princeton University Office of Population Research and the Association of Reproductive Health Professionals)
Tel: 888-NOT-2-LATE
Web: www.not-2-late.com

Go Ask Alice! (by Columbia University Health Education Program)
Lerner Hall
2920 Broadway, 7th Floor
MC 2608
New York, NY 10027
Tel: (212) 854-5453
Fax: (212) 854-8949
Web: www.goaskalice.columbia.edu

National Women's Health Information Center (by DHHS Office on Women's Health)
8550 Arlington Boulevard, Suite 300
Fairfax, VA 22031
Tel: 800-994-WOMAN
Web: www.4.woman.org

The Society of Obstetricians and Gynecologists of Canada
780 Echo Drive
Ottawa ON
Canada K15 5R7
Tel: (613) 730-4192; 800-561-2416
Fax: (613) 730-4314
Web: www.sexualityandu.ca

STD Info Line
American Social Health Association
PO Box 13827
Research Triangle Park, NC 27709
Tel: 800-227-8922; 800-342-2437; 800-344-7432 (Spanish); 800-243-7889 (TTY service)
Web: www.ashastd.org; www.iwannaknow.org (for teens)

Teenwire (by Planned Parenthood Federation of America)
810 Seventh Avenue
New York, NY 10019
Tel: (212) 541-7800
Fax: (212) 245-1845
Web: www.teenwire.com

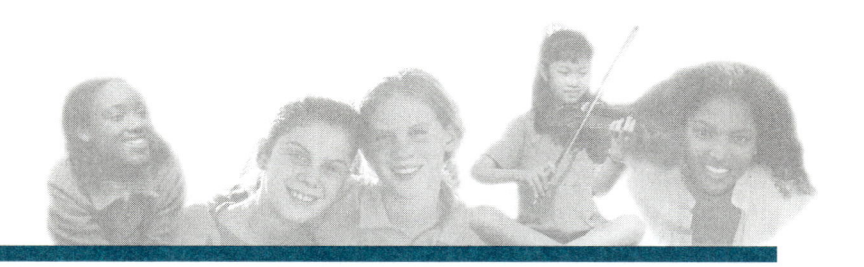

Condom Availability for Adolescents

KEY POINTS

➤ Although abstinence is the most effective way to avoid sexually transmitted disease (STD) infections and pregnancy, use of the latex condom should be promoted for sexually active adolescents. Condoms prevent the transmission of the human immunodeficiency virus (HIV) and can reduce the risks of other STDs.

➤ Adolescents must be taught to use condoms properly and consistently. Confusion about the correct way to use condoms is common among adolescents.

➤ Adolescents face many obstacles to obtaining and using condoms, including confidentiality, cost, access, transportation, embarrassment, and objection by a partner.

➤ Condoms should be available through various channels, including families, medical facilities, commercial channels, and schools. Making condoms available at schools can increase condom use among sexually active students but does not increase sexual activity.

➤ Adolescents who have discussed condoms and STD infection with their parents or health care providers are more likely to use condoms than those who have not.

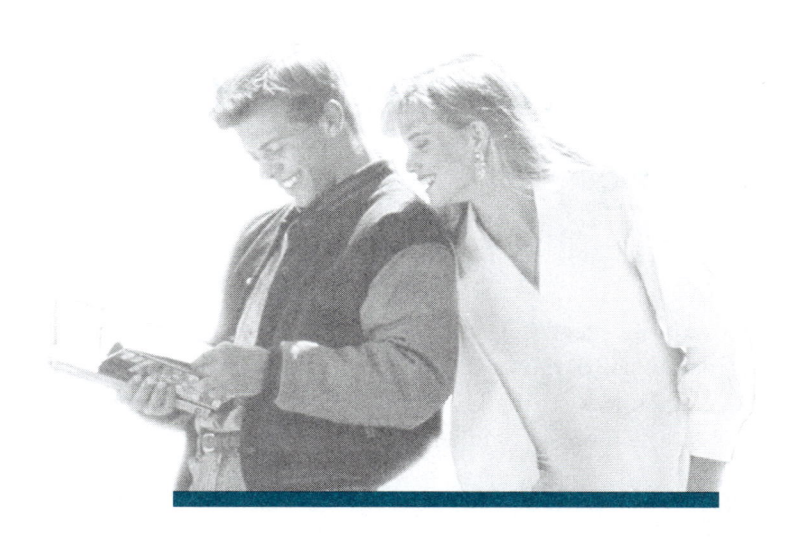

Nationwide, 46% of all high-school students report having sexual intercourse. In addition, 7% of these students had initiated sexual intercourse before age 13 years. Approximately 14% of all sexually active students report having had four or more partners (1).

The health consequences of unprotected intercourse among adolescents have been shown through the high rates of adolescent pregnancy and sexually transmitted diseases (STDs) in the United States. Despite similar rates of sexual activity, the United States has the highest adolescent pregnancy rate of any Western developed country (2). Each year, between 800,000 to 900,000 women aged 15–19 years become pregnant (3). Nearly four million new STD infections occur each year among adolescents. This accounts for roughly one quarter of the 15 million new STD infections that occur annually in the United States (4). Sexually transmitted disease infection rates tend to be higher for females than for males. This discrepancy can be attributed partially to the focus of screening programs on females that result in a lack of identification of males with STDs. Also, many STDs are transmitted more efficiently from males to females than from females to males. Females aged 15–19 years have the highest rates of chlamydia infection among individuals of all ages (5). Even with the overall decreases in gonorrhea rates, adolescents aged 15–19 years had the highest age-specific gonorrhea rates among females and the third highest rates among males in 2001 (5). Most notably, the number of individuals aged 13–19 years with cases of acquired immunodeficiency syndrome (AIDS) has increased from one case in 1981 to 4,428 cases in 2001; 322 of these cases were newly diagnosed during 2001 (6).

Effectiveness of Condoms in Preventing Sexually Transmitted Diseases and Pregnancy

Abstinence is the most effective way for adolescents to avoid STDs and pregnancy. Use of latex condoms should be promoted for sexually active adolescents as the only device currently available to reduce the risk of human immunodeficiency virus (HIV) infections and STDs (7). Latex condoms also protect against unintended pregnancy. Understating condom efficacy weakens counseling and inappropriately discourages their use.

Understating condom efficacy weakens counseling and inappropriately discourages their use.

According to the Centers for Disease Control and Prevention, latex condoms, when used consistently and correctly, are highly effective in preventing the transmission of HIV and can reduce the risks of other STDs, including chlamydia, gonorrhea, and trichomoniasis (8). They also can reduce the risk of genital herpes, syphilis, chancroid, and human papillomavirus infection when the infected areas are covered or protected by the condom (8). In addition, the use of latex condoms has been associated with a reduction in the risk of human papillomavirus-associated diseases, such as cervical cancer (8). Natural membrane condoms are not as protective as latex condoms (9). There is as yet inadequate data on the use of the female condom by adolescents.

Many young women want to prevent pregnancy with a method that is completely within their control, and a number of such methods are available, such as hormonal methods. It is important, however, to educate adolescent males and females who depend on hormonal methods of contraception that these methods do not prevent HIV or other STDs. Although dual use may be perceived as more difficult to maintain than reliance on a single method, condom use must be promoted in conjunction with other contraceptive methods, as well as on its own. In addition, because the risk of STDs increases with exposure to multiple partners, adolescents who are sexually active also should be encouraged to limit their number of sexual partners and to use condoms, even if they only have one sexual partner at that time. It is important to note that although many adolescents may say that they have only one sexual partner, they change partners frequently, which increases their risk for STDs.

Condoms are 97% effective in preventing pregnancy if used correctly and consistently (10). One study that compared the relative effectiveness of contraceptive methods in actual use showed that only 15% of women using male condoms experienced contraceptive failure during the first 12 months of use, compared with 85% of those using no method and 21–26% of those using methods such as periodic abstinence or spermicide alone. Contraceptive failure rates vary more by user characteristics, such as marital status, income, race and ethnicity, and age, than by method. Among female adolescents, condom failure rates range from 12.6% for those who are married to 31% for those who are unmarried but cohabit (11).

Condom failure rates can be attributed primarily to improper and inconsistent use rather than manufacturing defects or breakage (9). In the United States, the condom breakage rate during use ranges from 0.4% to 2.3%, most of which results from incorrect use rather than poor quality (7, 9). In addition to quality assurance methods used by manufacturers, condoms are regulated by the U.S. Food and Drug Administration and tested for resistance to breakage and leaks, which reduces the risk of selling defective condoms (7). In the rare event of condom failure, emergency contraception should be easily accessible.

Condom failure rates can be attributed primarily to improper and inconsistent use rather than manufacturing defects or breakage...

Factors Affecting Condom Use

Overall, increases in condom use can be seen among adolescents nationwide. Reported condom use at last intercourse for all sexually active high-school students has increased from 46% in 1991 to 58% in 2001 (1). However, high rates of unintended pregnancy and STDs in the United States suggest the sporadic use of condoms and other contraceptives among sexually active adolescents, as well as adults. Approximately 32% of sexually active 15–17 year olds and 34% of sexually active 18–19 year olds reported use of condoms as their current contraception method (12). All age groups, including adolescents, can improve their use of condoms.

Adolescents trade off between hormonal contraceptives and condoms according to partner type and perceived risks of pregnancy and STD acquisition. Both females and males reported less condom use and more hormonal contraceptive use with main partners than with casual partners (32). To increase the likelihood of simultaneous use of both methods, health care providers should tailor counseling to the adolescent patient's perceived risk of STDs and pregnancy and stress that the best way to prevent both is to use hormonal methods and condoms.

Sexually active adolescents, male and female, must be taught to use condoms properly, effectively, and consistently. Successful condom use requires using a new condom for each act of intercourse; putting it on correctly (leaving some room at the tip) before penetration; withdrawing while the penis is still erect, holding the condom firmly while withdrawing the penis to keep it from slipping off; and using only water-based lubricants, not those that are oil-based, such as petroleum jelly, shortening, mineral oil, massage oils, body lotions, or cooking oil (13). Confusion about the correct way to use condoms is common among adolescents and often leads to the following mistakes: 1) no space being left at the tip of the condom; 2) using petroleum jelly with condoms; and 3) thinking nonlatex condoms protect against AIDS better than latex condoms (14). In addition, young women must learn to communicate the need for condom use to their sexual partners, a skill that is not easy in practice even for older, more experienced women. Adolescents are more likely to use condoms if they (15–19):

- Receive comprehensive HIV and AIDS education
- Believe that condoms can prevent HIV infection
- Perceive peer norms as supporting condom use
- Are not embarrassed to be asked by a partner to use condoms
- Carry condoms with them
- Have discussed HIV and AIDS with a physician
- Have easy access to condoms
- Have a partner who is similar in age, grade, or school
- Have the decisiveness and verbal skills needed to ask a partner to use condoms

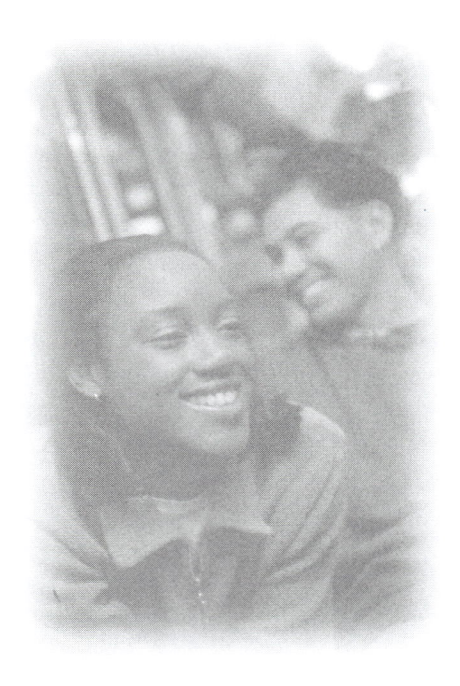

Overcoming Barriers to Condom Use

Adolescents face many obstacles to obtaining and using condoms. Some of these obstacles relate to confidentiality, cost, access, transportation, embarrassment, objection by a partner, perception that it is easy to determine whether or not a partner has an STD or has had multiple partners, and the perception that the risks of pregnancy and infection are low (15–20). Although condoms are a widely available nonprescription item, this does not necessarily translate into ready access for adolescents. For example, in a 1996 survey of drugstores and convenience stores by adolescents in Washington, DC, only 33% of the stores clearly indicated where condoms were shelved. Condoms were kept behind a counter in 83% of all convenience stores and 15% of drug stores, necessitating assistance from a store clerk (21). This result is consistent with a new study indicating that the majority of private grocery stores and convenience stores kept condoms behind the counter (82% and 56%, respectively) (22). Furthermore, adolescent females asking for help in finding and purchasing condoms reported encountering "resistance or condemnation" 27% of the time (21).

Eliminating barriers to the use of condoms and establishing condom use as the norm for sexually active adolescents will help adolescents protect themselves. Discussions about condoms between parents and adolescents that occur before sexual initiation are associated with greater condom use during the first and most recent intercourse and use of condoms during 50% of sexual encounters (23). Health care providers also play an important role in condom use. Adolescents who have discussed HIV infection with a physician are 1.7 times more likely to use condoms than those who have not (18).

One of the more controversial approaches to increase condom use among adolescents is making condoms available in schools. Much of the debate about condom availability programs has been ideologic; it has not focused on condom effectiveness or program effectiveness (24). For example, one major objection is that providing condoms will promote sexual activity, yet there is no evidence to indicate that this is true (25). Despite the controversy, a Gallup poll taken in August 1992 found that 68% of 1,316 adults surveyed thought condoms should be available in the schools, and a separate survey of 2,100 high-school seniors showed that 81% felt condoms should be available in schools. Seventy-eight percent of these same students felt condom availability did not encourage sexual activity (26, 27).

Several studies indicate that condom availability programs do not increase sexual activity. A study of New York City's school condom availability program found a significant increase in condom use among sexually active students, but no increase in sexual activity (28). Likewise, a study of Philadelphia health resource centers that dispense condoms did not show an increase in sexually active adolescents; rather, the study did suggest a decrease in the number of students ever having intercourse. In addition, the percentage of sexually active students who reported using condoms at last intercourse increased from 52% to 58% (29). A study of condom availability in Seattle schools showed no increase in sexual activity. There was no effect on condom (or birth control pill) use in schools where condoms were made available only in vending machines, but schools with both school clinics and condom vending machines showed decreased condom use, which was offset by increased birth control pill use (30). Overall, students in high schools, alternative schools, or small schools with condom-availability programs; schools that allow condoms to be easily accessible in baskets or bowls; or schools that make them available through school health centers obtained higher levels of condom use by students than those in other schools (31).

Summary

Abstinence should be stressed as the only certain way to prevent STDs and pregnancy. Because the majority of adolescents do become sexually active, both male and female adolescents also must be taught to use condoms properly, effectively, and consistently. The latex condom should be made widely available to adolescents. Studies have consistently shown that doing so will not increase sexual activity. Ideally, adolescents should have access to condom education and counseling when contraception is dispensed. However, condoms should be made easily available. Condoms should be available not only through families, medical facilities, and commercial channels, but also through other appropriate and informed individuals, without cost if possible, at sites where adolescents congregate. These sites may include schools, clubs, and other agencies serving adolescents. A clear message from the medical community supporting condom use will enhance the prevention of STDs and unintended pregnancy.

References

1. Grunbaum JA, Kann L, Kinchen SA, Williams B, Ross JG, Lowry R, et al. Youth risk behavior surveillance—United States, 2001. MMWR Surveill Summ 2002;51(4):1–62.
2. Singh S, Darroch JE. Adolescent pregnancy and childbearing: levels and trends in developed countries. Fam Plann Perspect 2000;32:14–23.
3. Ventura SJ, Mosher WD, Curtin SC, Abma JC, Henshaw S. Trends in pregnancy rates for the United States, 1976-97: an update. Natl Vital Stat Rep 2001;49(4):1–9.
4. American Social Health Association. Sexually transmitted diseases in America: how many cases and at what cost? Menlo Park (CA): Kaiser Family Foundation; 1998. Available at http://www.kff.org/content/archive/1445/std_rep.pdf. Retrieved October 16, 2002.
5. Centers for Disease Control and Prevention. Sexually transmitted disease surveillance, 2001. Atlanta (GA): CDC; 2002.
6. Centers for Disease Control and Prevention. HIV/AIDS surveillance report. 2001;13(2):1–48.

7. Sexually transmitted diseases treatment guidelines 2002. Centers for Disease Control and Prevention. MMWR 2002:51(RR-6):1–78.
8. Male latex condoms and sexually transmitted diseases: fact sheet for public health personnel. Atlanta (GA): Centers for Disease Control and Prevention; 2003. Available at http://www.cdc.gov/hiv/pubs/facts/condoms.pdf. Retrieved February 3, 2003.
9. Frezieres RG, Walsh TL, Nelson AL, Clark VA, Coulson AH. Evaluation of the efficacy of a polyurethane condom: results from a randomized, controlled clinical trial. Fam Plann Perspect 1999;31:81–7.
10. Hatcher RA, Trussell J, Stewart F, Cates W Jr, Stewart GK, Guest F, et al. Contraceptive technology. 17th revised ed. New York: Ardent Media; 1998.
11. Fu H, Darroch JE, Haas T, Ranjit N. Contraceptive failure rates: new estimates from the 1995 National Survey of Family Growth. Fam Plann Perspect 1999;31:56–63.
12. Bankole A, Darroch JE, Singh S. Determinants of trends in condom use in the United States, 1988–1995. Fam Plann Perspect 1999;31:264–71.
13. Update: barrier protection against HIV infection and other sexually transmitted diseases. MMWR Morb Mortal Wkly Rep 1993;42:589–91, 597.
14. Crosby RA, Yarber WL. Perceived versus actual knowledge about correct condom use among U.S. adolescents: results from a national study. J Adolesc Health 2001;28:415–20.
15. Rickert VI, Gottleib A, Jay S. A comparison of three clinic-based AIDS education programs on female adolescents' knowledge, attitudes, and behavior. J Adolesc Health Care 1990;11:298–303.
16. Ford K, Sohn W, Lepkowski J. Characteristics of adolescents' sexual partners and their association with use of condoms and other contraceptive methods. Fam Plann Perspect 2001; 33:100–5, 132.
17. Kegeles SM, Adler NE, Irwin CE Jr. Adolescents and condoms. Associations of beliefs with intentions to use. Am J Dis Child 1989;143:911–5.
18. Hingson RW, Strunin L, Berlin BM, Heeren T. Beliefs about AIDS, use of alcohol and drugs, and unprotected sex among Massachusetts adolescents. Am J Public Health 1990;80:295–9.
19. Baele J, Dusseldorp E, Maes S. Condom use self-efficacy: effect on intended and actual condom use in adolescents. J Adolesc Health 2001;28:421–31.
20. Siegel D, Lazarus N, Krasnovsky F, Durbin M, Chesney M. AIDS knowledge, attitudes, and behavior among inner city, junior high school students. J Sch Health 1991;61:160–65.
21. 1996 update of teens' survey of stores in the District of Columbia on accessibility of family planning methods. Washington, DC: Advocates for Youth; 1996.
22. Klein J, Rossbach C, Nijher H, Geist M, Wilson K, Cohn S, et al. Where do adolescents get their condoms? J Adolesc Health 2001;29:186–93.
23. Miller KS, Levin ML, Whitaker DJ, Xu X. Patterns of condom use among adolescents: the impact of mother-adolescent communication. Am J Public Health 1998;88:1542–4.
24. Samuels SE, Smith MD, eds. Condoms in the schools. Menlo Park (CA): The Henry J. Kaiser Family Foundation; 1993.
25. Kirby D. Emerging answers: research findings on programs to reduce teen pregnancy. Washington, DC: National Campaign to Prevent Teen Pregnancy; 2001.
26. Examiner News Service. Most in poll want condoms handed out. San Francisco Examiner 1992 Aug 28; Sect A13.
27. Peterson KS. Teen poll reveals AIDS fear. USA Today 1992 Apr 24; Sect 1D.
28. Guttmacher S, Lieberman L, Ward D, Freudenberg N, Radosh A, Des Jarlais D. Condom availability in New York City public high schools: relationships to condom use and sexual behavior. Am J Public Health 1997;87:1427–33.

29. Furstenberg FF Jr, Geitz LM, Teitler JO, Weiss CC. Does condom availability make a difference? An evaluation of Philadelphia's health resource centers. Fam Plann Perspect 1997;29:123–7.
30. Kirby D, Brener ND, Brown NL, Peterfreund N, Hillard P, Harrist R. The impact of condom availability in Seattle schools on sexual behavior and condom use. Am J Public Health 1999;89:182–7.
31. Kirby DB, Brown NL. Condom availability programs in U.S. schools. Fam Plann Perspect 1996;28:196–202.
32. Ott MA, Adler NE, Millstein SG, Tschann JM, Ellen JM. The trade-off between hormonal contraceptives and condoms among adolescents. Perspect Sex Reprod Health 2002;34:6–14.

Resources

ACOG Resources

American College of Obstetricians and Gynecologists. Anticoncepción. ACOG Patient Education Pamphlet SP005. Washington, DC: ACOG; 2000.

American College of Obstetricians and Gynecologists. Barrier methods of contraception. ACOG Patient Education Pamphlet AP022. Washington, DC: ACOG; 1999.

American College of Obstetricians and Gynecologists. Birth control. ACOG Patient Education Pamphlet AP005. Washington, DC: ACOG; 1999.

American College of Obstetricians and Gynecologists. Birth control—especially for teens. ACOG Patient Education Pamphlet AP112. Washington, DC: ACOG; 1997.

American College of Obstetricians and Gynecologists. Cómo prevenir enfermedades de transmisión sexual. ACOG Patient Education Pamphlet SP009. Washington, DC: ACOG; 1999.

American College of Obstetricians and Gynecologists. How to prevent sexually transmitted diseases. ACOG Patient Education Pamphlet AP009. Washington, DC: ACOG; 1999.

American College of Obstetricians and Gynecologists. Strategies for adolescent pregnancy prevention. Washington, DC: ACOG; 2002.

American College of Obstetricians and Gynecologists. Tool kit for teen care. Washington, DC: ACOG; 2003.

Other Resources

The following lists are for information purposes only. Referral to these sources and web sites does not imply the endorsement of ACOG. These lists are not meant to be comprehensive. The exclusion of a source or web site does not reflect the quality of that source or web site. Please note that web sites are subject to change without notice.

Advocates for Youth
1025 Vermont Avenue NW, Suite 200
Washington, DC 20005
Tel: (202) 347-5700
Fax: (202) 347-2263
Web: www.advocatesforyouth.org

American Academy of Family Physicians
11400 Tomahawk Creek Parkway
Leawood, KS 66211-2672
Tel: (913) 906-6000
Web: www.aafp.org

American Academy of Pediatrics
141 Northwest Point Boulevard
Elk Grove Village, IL 60007-1098
Tel: (847) 228-5005
Fax: (847) 228-5097
Web: www.aap.org

Society for Adolescent Medicine
1916 NW Copper Oaks Circle
Blue Springs, MO 64015
Tel: (816) 224-8010
Web: www.adolescenthealth.org

Resources for Your Patients

Advocates for Youth
1025 Vermont Avenue NW, Suite 200
Washington, DC 20005
Tel: (202) 347-5700
Fax: (202) 347-2263
Web: www.advocatesforyouth.org

Center for Young Women's Health
Children's Hospital
333 Longwood Avenue, 5th floor
Boston, MA 02115
Tel: (617) 355-CYWH (2994)
Fax: (617) 232-3136
Web: www.youngwomenshealth.org

Go Ask Alice! (by Columbia University Health Education Program)
Lerner Hall
2920 Broadway, 7th Floor
MC 2608
New York, NY 10027
Tel: (212) 854-5453
Fax: (212) 854-8949
Web: www.goaskalice.columbia.edu

National Women's Health Information Center (by DHHS Office on Women's Health)
8550 Arlington Boulevard, Suite 300
Fairfax, VA 22031
Tel: 800-994-WOMAN
Web: www.4woman.org

Teenwire (by Planned Parenthood Federation of America)
810 Seventh Avenue
New York, NY 10019
Tel: (212) 541-7800
Fax: (212) 245-1845
Web: www.teenwire.com

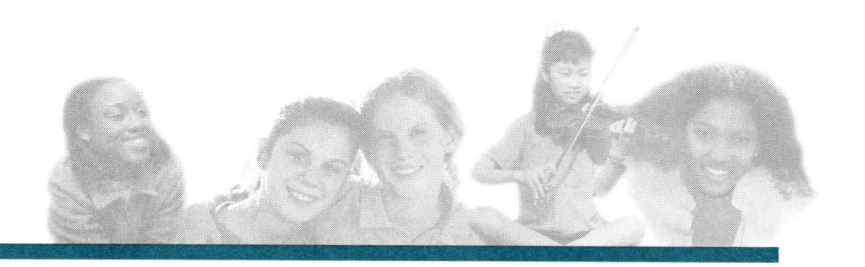

Adolescents' Right to Refuse Long-term Contraceptives

Key points

➢ Parents, health care agencies, social workers, and other guardians may request that long-term contraceptives be administered to adolescent girls against their wishes. The physician, however, should acknowledge that the adolescent is the patient who makes the final decision and has the right of free choice.

➢ Physicians should be aware that the adolescent patient has a right to privacy and to make reproductive decisions. Physicians should have knowledge of the state and local statutes regarding minors' rights in health care.

➢ The physician should assist the adolescent in the selection and use of an appropriate long-term or short-term contraceptive method to prevent pregnancy and sexually transmitted diseases.

➢ The physician should assess the reasons for the adult's request for long-term contraceptives for the adolescent patient. If a deep long-standing conflict between the adult and the adolescent exists, or in the case of the impaired adolescent, a referral to or involvement of an appropriate practitioner or agency may be necessary.

➢ Physicians should be available to address health concerns of adolescents and encourage parents to be supportive of the adolescents' growth and their responsibility for their own health care.

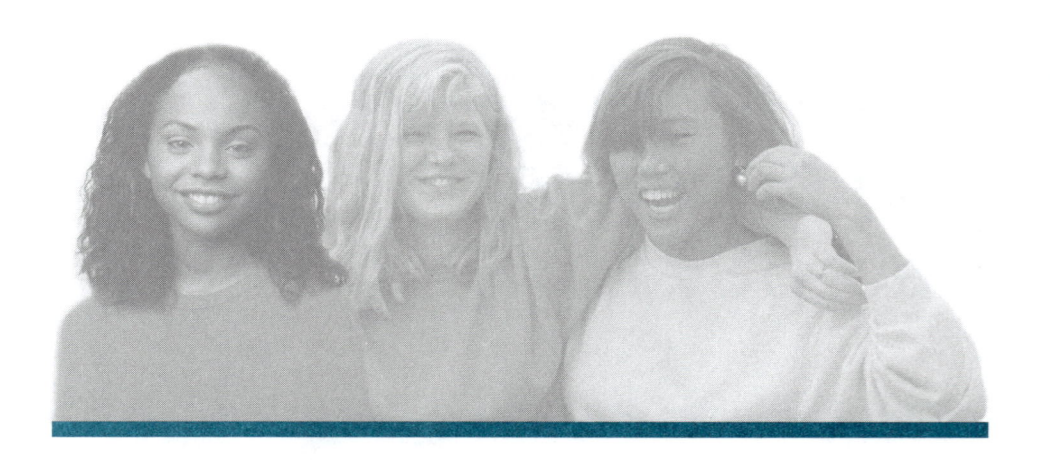

Long-acting progestin-only contraceptives are now readily available, and they are being widely promoted for use in women, including adolescents who will not or cannot use other contraceptive methods. The implantable and injectable progestins also are viewed by some individuals as a method of limiting adolescent pregnancies. This raises concerns about the adolescent's right to accept or refuse a method of contraception against parental request and about the potential coercive use of such contraceptives in minors.

Parents who feel their adolescent daughter is at risk for an unintended pregnancy may request that the physician administer long-term contraceptives to their daughter against her wishes. Health care agencies, social workers, and guardians may make similar requests. The physician, however, should acknowledge that the adolescent is the patient and has the final decision and right of free choice (1). Therefore, the adolescent has the right to refuse any method of contraception and to discontinue contraceptives—which includes removal of contraceptive implants—without parental notification or consent. (See "Confidentiality in Adolescent Health Care" chapter for more on minors' rights and confidentiality issues.)

Physicians providing care should have knowledge of their state laws regarding minors' rights and also should be aware that adolescents have constitutional rights to privacy and to make reproductive decisions. The U.S. Supreme Court first ruled more than 35 years ago that the Fourteenth Amendment protects the rights of minors as well as those of adults (2). The rights of minors are subject to more limitations than the rights of adults; however, a subsequent ruling held that minors have a constitutional right to privacy that includes the right to obtain contraceptives (3). Furthermore, as of this printing, laws in 27 states and the District of Columbia give minors the right to make informed decisions about contraceptives without parental involvement (4). There are no state laws that require parental involvement for a minor to obtain medical care in connection with contraceptive services (4).

The role of the physician in providing care to an adolescent is more than that of a technician who administers a contraceptive method. In the situation in which an adolescent refuses long-term contraceptives, the physician should explore thoroughly the reasons for her refusal (5). This process may help correct misinformation and allay fears. If the adolescent persists in

The role of the physician in providing care to an adolescent is more than that of a technician who administers a contraceptive method.

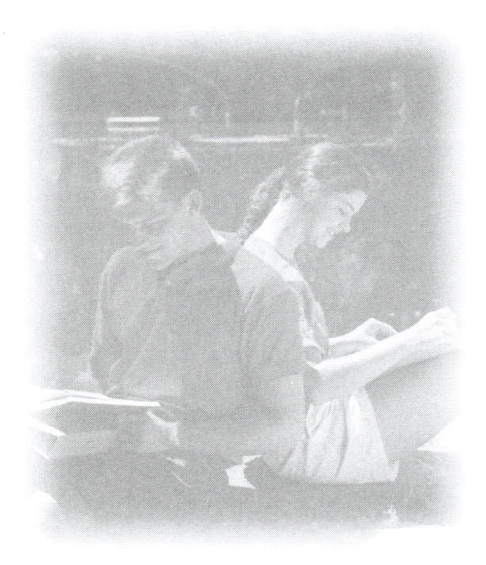

rejecting the long-term contraceptive method, the physician should assist her in the selection and correct consistent use of an appropriate reliable method to prevent pregnancy. Information also should be provided on how to avoid sexually transmitted diseases, including human immunodeficiency virus (HIV) infection, with both short- and long-term contraceptive methods.

The physician also should assess the reasons for the adult's request so that appropriate intervention can be instituted. If the physician determines or suspects that the disagreement between the minor and adult, especially parent or guardian, over a contraceptive choice reflects a deeper or more long-standing conflict, the physician may make a referral to an appropriate practitioner or agency. If the parent or guardian is requesting long-term contraception for an adolescent who is incapable of giving informed consent, the decision to use long-term contraception should be based on a careful assessment. This may involve a multidisciplinary team that includes an advocate appointed for the impaired adolescent.

Finally, regardless of whether an adolescent selects or refuses a long-term contraceptive method, the physician should remain available to address related health concerns. This includes a commitment to offer continuing contraceptive care, periodic evaluation for sexually transmitted diseases, and screening via a Pap test. Physicians should inform parents that it is appropriate for their maturing adolescents to assume increasing responsibility for their own health care and assist parents in guiding their daughters toward healthy development.

References

1. Confidential health services for adolescents. Council on Scientific Affairs, American Medical Association. JAMA 1993;269:1420–4.
2. In re Gault, 387 U.S. 1 (1967).
3. Carey, Governor of New York v. Population Services International, 431 U.S. 678 (1977).
4. Alan Guttmacher Institute. State policies in brief. Minors' access to contraceptive services. New York: AGI; 2002. Available at http://www.agi-usa.org/pubs/spib_MACS.pdf. Retrieved December 30, 2002.
5. Moreno JD. Treating the adolescent patient. An ethical analysis. J Adolesc Health Care 1989;10:454–9.

Resources

ACOG Resources

American College of Obstetricians and Gynecologists. Anticoncepción. ACOG Patient Education Pamphlet SP005. Washington, DC: ACOG; 2000.

American College of Obstetricians and Gynecologists. Birth control. ACOG Patient Education Pamphlet AP005. Washington, DC: ACOG; 1999.

American College of Obstetricians and Gynecologists. Birth control—especially for teens. ACOG Patient Education Pamphlet AP112. Washington, DC: ACOG; 1997.

American College of Obstetricians and Gynecologists. Ethics in obstetrics and gynecology. Washington, DC: ACOG; 2002.

American College of Obstetricians and Gynecologists. Tool kit for teen care. Washington, DC: ACOG; 2003.

OTHER RESOURCES

The following lists are for information purposes only. Referral to these sources and web sites does not imply the endorsement of ACOG. These lists are not meant to be comprehensive. The exclusion of a source or web site does not reflect the quality of that source or web site. Please note that web sites are subject to change without notice.

Alan Guttmacher Institute
120 Wall Street, 21st Floor
New York, NY 10005
Tel: (212) 248-1111
Fax: (212) 248-1952
Web: www.agi-usa.org

American Academy of Family Physicians
11400 Tomahawk Creek Parkway
Leawood, KS 66211-2672
Tel: (913) 906-6000
Web: www.aafp.org

American Academy of Pediatrics
141 Northwest Point Boulevard
Elk Grove Village, IL 60007-1098
Tel: (847) 434-4000
Fax: (847) 434-8000
Web: www.aap.org

American Medical Association
515 North State Street
Chicago, IL 60610
Tel: (312) 464-5000
Web: www.ama-assn.org

Center for Adolescent Health and the Law
211 North Columbia Street
Chapel Hill, NC 27514
Tel: (919) 968-8870
Fax: (919) 968-8854
Web: www.adolescenthealthlaw.org

Society for Adolescent Medicine
1916 NW Copper Oaks Circle
Blue Springs, MO 64015
Tel: (816) 224-8010
Web: www.adolescenthealth.org

RESOURCES FOR YOUR PATIENTS

Center for Young Women's Health
Children's Hospital
333 Longwood Avenue, 5th floor
Boston, MA 02115
Tel: (617) 355-CYWH (2994)
Fax: (617) 232-3136
Web: www.youngwomenshealth.org

Go Ask Alice! (by Columbia University Health Education Program)
Lerner Hall
2920 Broadway, 7th Floor
MC 2608
New York, NY 10027
Tel: (212) 854-5453
Fax: (212) 854-8949
Web: www.goaskalice.columbia.edu

National Women's Health Information Center (by DHHS Office on Women's Health)
8550 Arlington Boulevard, Suite 300
Fairfax, VA 22031
Tel: 800-994-WOMAN
Web: www.4woman.org

Teenwire (by Planned Parenthood Federation of America)
810 Seventh Avenue
New York, NY 10019
Tel: (212) 541-7800
Fax: (212) 245-1845
Web: www.teenwire.com

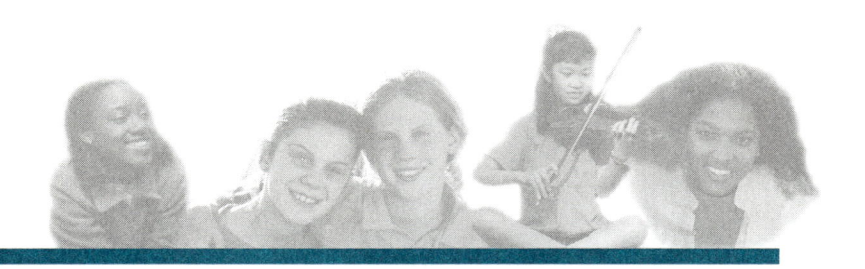

Screening for Chlamydia and Gonorrhea in Adolescents

Key points

- Chlamydia and gonorrhea are highly prevalent in adolescents, particularly in the southern region of the United States. However, their true incidence and prevalence are unknown.

- All sexually active adolescents should be screened for chlamydia and gonorrhea infections routinely. It also may be advisable to screen for these sexually transmitted diseases when they or their partners have new sexual partners.

- Urine screening should be considered when adolescents are reluctant to have pelvic examinations or are seen where pelvic examinations are not feasible.

- Ligase chain reaction is one of the nucleic acid amplification techniques used to test urine for chlamydia and gonorrhea.

- Endocervical specimens should be obtained in sexually active or symptomatic adolescents where pelvic examinations can and should be performed and also may be required in cases of alleged sexual assault.

- Although urine ligase chain reaction is more sensitive and almost as specific as cultures in screening and testing for chlamydia and gonorrhea, the latter may be less expensive and, therefore, more appropriate.

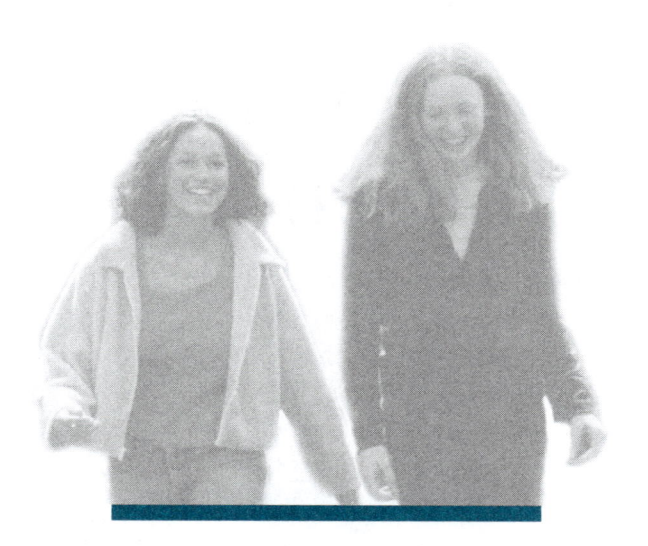

Sexually transmitted diseases (STDs) are a major health issue for adolescents. In the United States each year, nearly four million adolescents become infected with STDs. Adolescents account for approximately 25% of all new cases of STDs reported annually in the United States (1). Of reported cases of chlamydia in females in 2001, 40% were in those aged 15–19 years. Of reported cases of gonorrhea in females in 2001, 38% were in those aged 15–19 years, representing the highest age-specific chlamydia and gonorrhea rates among females (2). Because approximately 80% of chlamydia and 50% of gonorrhea cases are asymptomatic in women (3, 4), the true incidence and prevalence of these STDs are unknown and probably often are underreported.

It is difficult to identify appropriate populations to screen for gonorrhea and chlamydia. Identifying at-risk groups is only partially effective at detecting chlamydia and gonorrhea infections in sexually active adolescent females. Adolescents with multiple partners or prior history of an STD are considered at risk. However, several studies of sexually active adolescent girls failed to identify effective predictors of infections to specify a screening population (5–7). Obtaining an accurate history of at-risk behaviors in the adolescent population may be difficult because of denial, embarrassment, fear, mistrust, privacy concerns, as well as the real or perceived cultural attitude that looks down on adolescent females who are sexually active and may have an STD. The following factors need to be considered when recommending screening in adolescents:

- No studies give the actual prevalence or incidence of chlamydia or gonorrhea infections for the adolescent population.

- The incidence of reported chlamydia cases continues to increase each year, while the dramatic decrease in gonorrhea cases seen in the 1990s has leveled off (2).

- The highest prevalence of both chlamydia and gonorrhea as reported to the Centers for Disease Control and Prevention (CDC) occurs in the southern region of the United States (2). In this area, chlamydia may be approximately five times as common as gonorrhea (8), which has led to geographic variation in screening.

Adolescents account for approximately 25% of all new cases of STDs reported annually in the United States...

- At least one study reports an equal prevalence of chlamydia and gonorrhea in sexually active public high-school females in the mid-Atlantic states of approximately 15% (5).
- Although there may be a lower prevalence of chlamydia in private practice than in other settings (eg, STD clinics) (9), even a 2% prevalence in nulliparous females is significant in terms of the potential to spread disease and cause future reproductive health and infertility concerns.

The CDC has developed a computer program to help determine the cost-effectiveness of chlamydia screening (10).

Who Should be Screened for Chlamydia and Gonorrhea?

Because of the high prevalence of STDs in adolescents, their pathologic sequelae, and the high percentage of infections that are asymptomatic, screening programs are needed to identify and treat these diseases. Attention has been focused on chlamydia and gonorrhea because they are most prevalent in the adolescent population, are mostly asymptomatic, and are curable with antibiotics. Other STDs, such as herpes, hepatitis, and acquired immunodeficiency syndrome (AIDS), although of significance, are not currently curable. Emphasis must be placed on prevention. If a patient is diagnosed with an STD, she needs to be thoroughly screened for other STDs. In addition, it should be confirmed that she has been fully immunized against hepatitis B.

The American College of Obstetricians and Gynecologists recommends that providers annually screen for chlamydia and gonorrhea infection in all sexually active adolescents and other asymptomatic women at increased risk (11). The National Committee on Quality Assurance's Health Plan Employer Data and Information Set (HEDIS)* for managed care plans recommends annual routine testing for chlamydia in all sexually active women (12). Screening for chlamydia and gonorrhea currently is performed at the time of a pelvic examination. It may be advisable to rescreen patients if they or their partners have new sexual partners (6). According to the 1995 National Survey of Family Growth, 46% of women aged 15–19 years who had sex in the past year had two or more partners during the year (13). Given these data, approximately one half of adolescent females who are sexually active should be rescreened during any given year. However, rescreening is not consistently performed in this group. It is important for obstetrician–gynecologists to stress to all patients, but particularly adolescents, that rescreening with every partner change may be necessary. The CDC also recommends that all women with chlamydial infections, especially adolescents, be rescreened 3–4 months after treatment because of the high prevalence of reinfection (14).

---

*HEDIS is a set of standardized performance measures designed to ensure that purchasers and consumers have the information they need to reliably compare the performance of managed health care plans.

Urine Screening

Urine has been used effectively for several years to test for chlamydia and gonorrhea because the first 10 mL to 15 mL of voided urine will contain infected epithelial cells. Several types of tests exist (15). All methods use molecular biology to enzymatically duplicate and amplify specific nucleic acid sequences. Nucleic acid amplification techniques, such as ligase chain reaction, are designed to improve the sensitivity of assays based on nucleic acids.

Some adolescents are reluctant to have pelvic examinations as part of preventive health visits or are seen where pelvic examinations are not feasible. These factors reduce the capacity to screen for chlamydia and gonorrhea by endocervical specimen. Urine specimens should be considered for screening for chlamydia and gonorrhea and may be useful for group screening and identifying the prevalence of these diseases.

Ligase chain reaction is one of the tests most frequently studied. Ligase chain reaction technology is based on four oligonucleotide probes that recognize and hybridize to a specific target sequence within the organism being tested. Numerous studies in the United States and Europe have established the ligase chain reaction test for both endocervical specimen and urine as effective in both screening and selective testing. It is routinely more sensitive and specific than other forms of antigen and antibody testing (see Box 4). A representative study showed that in urine screening for chlamydia, ligase chain reaction has a sensitivity of 88.6%, specificity of 99.7%, and positive and negative predictive values of 96.9% and 99.0%, respectively, whereas the results for culture were 71.4%, 100%, 100%, and 97.6%, respectively (16). Thus, urine ligase chain reaction, being more sensitive and almost as specific as endocervical culture, may be the preferred test instead of ligase chain reaction culture performed on an endocervical swab specimen for chlamydia and gonorrhea. Although ligase chain reaction may cost more than cultures, laboratory costs vary (Table 2). A small percentage of tests may be falsely reported as negative because of inhibitors in the urine. This may be decreased by cooling or diluting the urine (17–20).

In sexually active or symptomatic adolescents where pelvic examinations can and should be performed, endocervical specimens should be obtained. Although urine ligase chain reaction may be more sensitive,

---

Box 4. Test Validity

Four measures of validity (the ability to differentiate between sick and well persons) describe test performance.

1. Sensitivity—The ability of a test to identify those who have the disease.
2. Specificity—The ability of a test to identify those who do not have the disease.
3. Predictive value positive—The likelihood that a person with a positive test has the disease.
4. Predictive value negative—The likelihood that a person with a negative test does not have the disease.

Reprinted with permission from Grimes D (ed). STD Update: Incidence Trends and New Screening Tests. The Contraception Report, 2000;11(3):7–8. Available at http://www.contraceptiononline.org/contrareport.

Table 2. Common Screening and Diagnostic Tests for *Neisseria Gonorrhoeae* and *Chlamydia Trachomatis* Genital Infections

Test Category	Test	Organism Tested	Usual Collection Site	Test May Be Performed By*	Cost†	Sensitivity	Specificity
Microscopy	Gram stain	Gonorrhea	Cervix, urethra	1, 2, 3, 4	$	Low	Low
	Giesma stain	Chlamydia	Cervix, urethra	1, 2, 3, 4	$	Low	Low
Culture	Thayer–Martin	Gonorrhea	Cervix, urethra	2, 3, 4, 5	$, $$	High	—
	Multiple cell lines	Chlamydia	Cervix, urethra	3, 4, 5	$$, $$$	High	Very high
Antigen tests, antibody tests	EIA, direct fluorescent antibody, nucleic acid probe hybridization	Gonorrhea, chlamydia	Cervix, urethra, urine	1, 2, 3, 4	$$, $$$	High	High
Nucleic acid amplification tests	PCR, ligase chain reaction, transcription mediated amplification, strand displacement amplification test	Gonorrhea, chlamydia	Cervix, urethra, urine	3, 4, 5	$$, $$$, $$$$	Very high	Very high

Abbreviations: EIA, enzyme based immunoassay; PCR, polymerase chain reaction.
*Testing places: 1, in physician's office or clinic; 2, in small hospital laboratory; 3, in large hospital laboratory; 4, in reference laboratory; 5, usually more than 2 days for results.
†Cost (highly variable by site): $, less than $10; $$, usually between $10 and $50; $$$, usually between $50 and $100; $$$$, may be more than $100.

cultures or immunoassays may be more appropriate because of cost constraints (15).

Sexual Assault

In cases of alleged sexual assault, endocervical or anorectal cultures may be needed for legal purposes, but urine ligase chain reaction or endocervical ligase chain reaction or both may be performed for improved detection of infections needing treatment. Because false negatives in cultures are not uncommon, a cervical or urine specimen for DNA testing may be appropriate in addition to, or instead of, cultures as determined by the examining physician on a case-by-case basis. In prepubertal children, however, DNA testing, including ligase chain reaction testing, is not appropriate for STD testing. At this time, only standard culture systems for the isolation of *Chlamydia trachomatis* and *Neisseria gonorrhoeae* are recommended for that population for legal purposes. Data are insufficient to adequately assess the utility of nucleic acid amplification tests in the evaluation of children who may have been sexually abused (14). Expert opinion suggests that these tests may be an alternative if culture systems for chlamydia are unavailable (14). It should be noted that in sexual abuse cases, a specificity as near 100% as possible is desirable to prevent false positive results (15). This degree of specificity is documented with cultures (16).

Summary

Chlamydia and gonorrhea infections are a significant health risk for adolescents and have long-term health consequences. It is difficult, however, to identify a specific high-risk adolescent population that can be targeted for screening. At a minimum, all sexually active adolescents should be tested routinely for gonorrhea and chlamydia. The National Committee on Quality Assurance's Health Plan Employer Data and Information Set defines routinely to be annually. It also may be advisable that sexually active adolescents and young women also should be tested when they or their partners have new partners. If universal screening of sexually active adolescents for chlamydia and gonorrhea is performed, the use of nucleic acid amplification testing on urine is recommended for adolescents who do not have pelvic examinations. All adolescents with positive test results for STDs on screening need to have follow-up for treatment, counseling about prevention, and a rescreening examination for reinfection 3–4 months after treatment. In addition, they need to be thoroughly screened for other STDs, and their hepatitis B immunization status should be reviewed. In cases of alleged sexual assault, endocervical or anorectal cultures are needed for legal purposes, but urine ligase chain reaction or endocervical ligase chain reaction or both may be performed for improved detection of infections.

References

1. Cates W Jr. Estimates of the incidence and prevalence of sexually transmitted diseases in the United States. American Social Health Association Panel. Sex Transm Dis 1999;26(suppl 4):S2–7.
2. Centers for Disease Control and Prevention. Sexually Transmitted Disease Surveillance 2001. Atlanta (GA): CDC; 2002.
3. National guideline for the management of Chlamydia trachomatis genital tract infection. Clinical Effectiveness Group, (Association of Genitourinary Medicine and the Medical Society for the Study of Venereal Diseases). Sex Transm Infect 1999;75:S4–8.

4. National guideline for the management of gonorrhea in adults. Clinical Effectiveness Group (Association of Genitourinary Medicine and the Medical Society for the Study of Venereal Diseases). Sex Transm Infect 1999;75:S13–5.

5. Burstein GR, Waterfield G, Joffe A, Zenilman JM, Quinn TC, Gaydos CA. Screening for gonorrhea and chlamydia by DNA amplification in adolescents attending middle school health centers. Opportunity for early intervention. Sex Transm Dis 1998;25:395–402.

6. Burstein GR, Gaydos CA, Diener-West M, Howell MR, Zenilman JM, Quinn TC. Incident Chlamydia trachomatis infections among inner-city adolescent females. JAMA 1998;280:521–6.

7. Mosure DJ, Berman S, Kleinbaum D, Halloran ME. Predictors of Chlamydia trachomatis infection among female adolescents: a longitudinal analysis. Am J Epidemiol 1996;144:997–1003.

8. Cohen DA, Nsuami M, Martin DH, Farley TA. Repeated school-based screening for sexually transmitted diseases: a feasible strategy for reaching adolescents. Pediatrics 1999;104:1281–5.

9. Best D, Ford CA, Miller WC. Prevalence of Chlamydia trachomatis and Neisseria gonorrhoeae infection in pediatric private practice. Pediatrics 2001;108:E103.

10. Centers for Disease Control and Prevention. Chlamydia screening, HEDIS and managed care. SOCRATES. Screening optimally for chlamydia: resource allocation, testing and evaluation software. Available at http://www.cdc.gov/nchstp/dstd/Software/socrates.htm. Retrieved December 27, 2002.

11. American College of Obstetricians and Gynecologists. Guidelines for Women's Health Care. 2nd ed. Washington, DC: ACOG; 2002.

12. National Committee for Quality Assurance. HEDIS 2001 Technical Specifications. Vol 2. Washington, DC: NCQA; 2000.

13. Finer LB, Darroch JE, Singh S. Sexual partnership patterns as a behavioral risk factor for sexually transmitted diseases. Fam Plann Perspect 1999;31: 228–36.

14. Sexually transmitted diseases treatment guidelines 2002. Centers for Disease Control and Prevention. MMWR Recomm Rep 2002;51(RR-6): 1–78.

15. Centers for Disease Control and Prevention. Screening tests to detect Chlamydia trachomatis and Neisseria gonorrhoeae infections—2002. MMWR 2002;51(No. RR-15):1–38.

16. Gaydos CA, Howell MR, Quinn TC, Gaydos JC, McKee KT Jr. Use of ligase chain reaction with urine versus cervical culture for detection of Chlamydia trachomatis in an asymptomatic military population of pregnant and non-pregnant females attending Papanicolaou smear clinics. J Clin Microbiol 1998;36:1300–4.

17. Berg ES. False-negative results of a ligase chain reaction assay to detect Chlamydia trachomatis due to inhibitors in urine. Eur J Clin Microbiol Infect Dis 1997;16:727–31.

18. Chernesky MA, Jang D, Sellors J, Luinstra K, Chong S, Castriciano S, et al. Urinary inhibitors of polymerase chain reaction and ligase chain reaction and testing of multiple specimens may contribute to lower assay sensitivities for diagnosing Chlamydia trachomatis infected women. Mol Cell Probes 1997;11:243–9.

19. Mahony J, Chong S, Jang D, Luinstra K, Faught M, Dalby D, et al. Urine specimens from pregnant and nonpregnant women inhibitory to amplification of Chlamydia trachomatis nucleic acid by PCR, ligase chain reaction, and transcription-mediated amplification: identification of urinary substances associ-

ated with inhibition and removal of inhibitory activity. J Clin Microbiol 1998;36:3122–6.
20. Moller JK, Anderson B, Olesen F, Lignell T, Ostergaard L. Impact of menstrual cycle on the diagnostic performance of LCR, TMA, and PCE for detection of Chlamydia trachomatis in home obtained and mailed vaginal flush and urine samples. Sex Transm Infect 1999;75:228–30.

Resources

ACOG Resources

American College of Obstetricians and Gynecologists. Cómo prevenir enfermedades de transmisión sexual. ACOG Patient Education Pamphlet SP009. Washington, DC: ACOG, 1999.

American College of Obstetricians and Gynecologists. Gonorrhea, chlamydia, and syphilis. ACOG Patient Education Pamphlet AP071. Washington, DC: ACOG; 2000.

American College of Obstetricians and Gynecologists. How to prevent sexually transmitted diseases. ACOG Patient Education Pamphlet AP009. Washington, DC: ACOG; 1999.

American College of Obstetricians and Gynecologists. Primary and preventive care: periodic assessments. ACOG Committee Opinion 246. Washington, DC: ACOG; 2000.

American College of Obstetricians and Gynecologists. Tool kit for teen care. Washington, DC: ACOG; 2003.

Other Resources

The following lists are for information purposes only. Referral to these sources and web sites does not imply the endorsement of ACOG. This list is not meant to be comprehensive. The exclusion of a source or web site does not reflect the quality of that source or web site. Please note that web sites are subject to change without notice.

American Academy of Family Physicians
11400 Tomahawk Creek Parkway
Leawood, KS 66211-2672
Tel: (913) 906-6000
Web: www.aafp.org

American Academy of Pediatrics
141 Northwest Point Boulevard
Elk Grove Village, IL 60007-1098
Tel: (847) 434-4000
Fax: (847) 434-8000
Web: www.aap.org

American Medical Association
515 North State Street
Chicago, IL 60610
Tel: (312) 464-5000
Web: www.ama-assn.org

American Social Health Association
PO Box 13827
Research Triangle Park, NC 27709
Tel: 800-227-8922; (919) 361-8400
Fax: (919) 361-8425
Web: www.ashastd.org

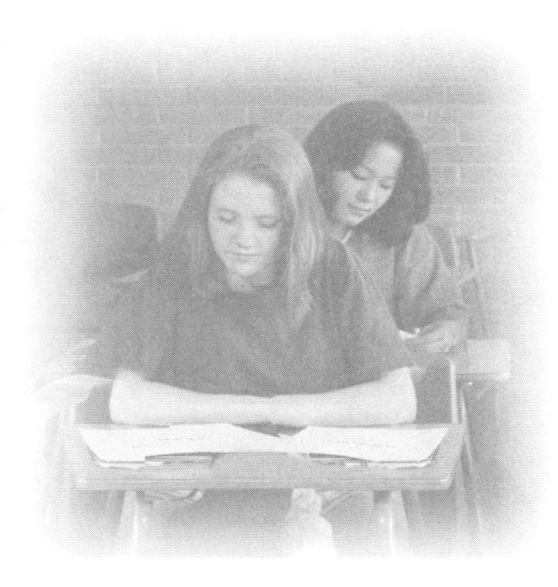

Centers for Disease Control and Prevention
National Center for Chronic Disease Prevention and Health Promotion
Division of Adolescent and School Health
4770 Buford Highway NE, Mail Stop K-32
Atlanta, GA 30341-3717
Tel: (770) 488-3168
Web: www.cdc.gov/nccdphp/dash/

Centers for Disease Control and Prevention
Office of Women's Health
600 Clifton Road, MS: D-51
Atlanta GA 30333
Tel: (404) 639-7230
Fax: (404) 639-7331

Planned Parenthood Federation of America, Inc.
810 Seventh Avenue
New York, NY 10019
Tel: (212) 541-7800
Fax: (212) 245-1845
Web: www.plannedparenthood.org

Society for Adolescent Medicine
1916 NW Copper Oaks Circle
Blue Springs, MO 64015
Tel: (816) 224-8010
Web: www.adolescenthealth.org

The Society of Obstetricians and Gynecologists of Canada
780 Echo Drive
Ottawa ON
Canada K15 5R7
Tel: (613) 730-4192; 800-561-2416
Fax: (613) 730-4314
Web: www.sexualityandu.ca

RESOURCES FOR YOUR PATIENTS

AWARE Foundation
1015 Chestnut Street, Suite 1225
Philadelphia, PA 19107-4302
Tel: (215) 955-9847
Web: www.awarefoundation.org

Center for Young Women's Health
Children's Hospital
333 Longwood Avenue, 5th floor
Boston, MA 02115
Tel: (617) 355-CYWH (2994)
Fax: (617) 232-3136
Web: www.youngwomenshealth.org

Go Ask Alice! (by Columbia University Health Education Program)
Lerner Hall
2920 Broadway, 7th Floor
MC 2608
New York, NY 10027
Tel: (212) 854-5453
Fax: (212) 854-8949
Web: www.goaskalice.columbia.edu

National Women's Health Information Center (by DHHS Office on Women's Health)
8550 Arlington Boulevard, Suite 300
Fairfax, VA 22031
Tel: 800-994-WOMAN
Web: www.4woman.org

The Society of Obstetricians and Gynecologists of Canada
780 Echo Drive
Ottawa ON
Canada K15 5R7
Tel: (613) 730-4192; 800-561-2416
Fax: (613) 730-4314
Web: www.sexualityandu.ca

STD Info Line
American Social Health Association
PO Box 13827
Research Triangle Park, NC 27709
Tel: 800-227-8922; 800-342-2437; 800-344-7432 (Spanish); 800-243-7889 (TTY service)
Web: www.ashastd.org; www.iwannaknow.org (for adolescents)

Teenwire (by Planned Parenthood Federation of America)
810 Seventh Avenue
New York, NY 10019
Tel: (212) 541-7800
Fax: (212) 245-1845
Web: www.teenwire.com

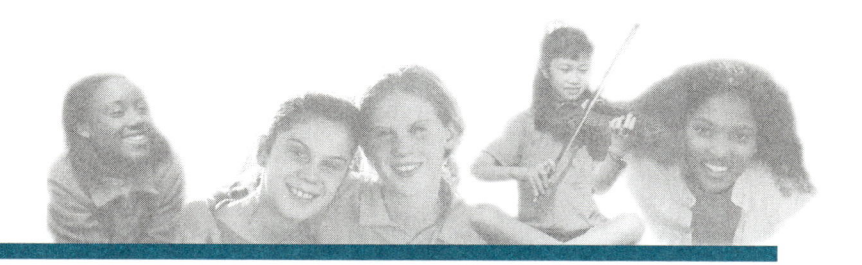

Eating Disorders

KEY POINTS

- It is estimated that five million Americans are affected yearly by eating disorders, including anorexia nervosa, bulimia nervosa, binge eating disorder, and female athlete triad.

- Anorexia is diagnosed if the patient refuses to maintain a minimally normal weight for age and height, has intense fear of gaining weight or being fat, exhibits undue influence of body weight or shape on self-image, denies the seriousness of the current low body weight, and has amenorrhea.

- Anorexia may lead to a number of serious health problems, including bone loss, osteoporosis, and death.

- A patient with bulimia consumes large amounts of food, frequently in secret, and then purges to compensate the caloric overload by vomiting, taking laxatives, fasting, and exercising to extremes. Patients with bulimia are more difficult to identify because their weight is typically normal to slightly above normal.

- Health consequences of bulimia include gastrointestinal disorders, pulmonary disorders, and death.

- Binge eating disorder is a variant of bulimia nervosa. A patient with binge eating disorder consumes large amounts of food, but does not purge to compensate for excessive food intakes.

- Many binge eaters are obese and experience attendant complications. Binge eating often is associated with depression.

- Female athlete triad refers to the inter-relatedness of eating disorders, amenorrhea, and osteoporosis that are associated with athletic training. The athletes who engage in sports in which a low body weight and lean physique are desired are at the greatest risk for female athlete triad.

- Patients with an eating disorder may manifest various presentations. The American College of Obstetricians and Gynecologists recommends that all adolescents be screened anually for eating disorders.

- It is important to assess the need for emergency admission of the patient with an eating disorder to the hospital because life-threatening conditions may arise.

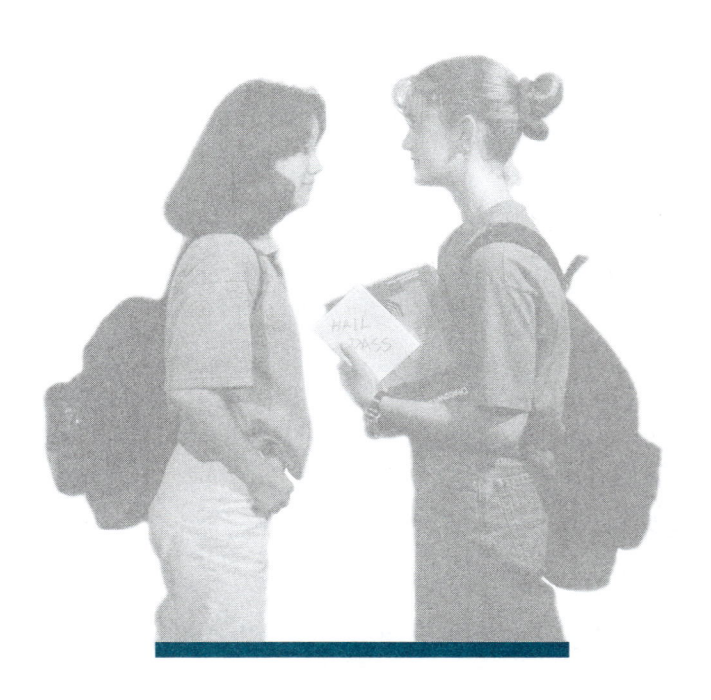

Every year, an estimated five million Americans are affected by eating disorders (1). Anorexia nervosa, bulimia nervosa, binge eating disorder, and the female athlete triad are thought to be the consequence of obsessive thoughts of thinness. Once limited to the affluent upper class, eating disorders no longer recognize socioeconomic, racial, and ethnic barriers (2). Anorexia is the third most common chronic disease following obesity and asthma among women between the ages of 15 and 19 years in the United States (3). Up to 20% of young women are affected by bulimia and the behavior frequently continues well into adulthood (4). Its actual incidence among older women is not known. Anorexia and bulimia often co-exist: almost one half of individuals with anorexia demonstrate bulimic behaviors and up to 80% of individuals with bulimia report a history of anorexia (5). There are no reliable population estimates for binge eating disorder, but it is thought to be at least as common as the other conditions combined (6). More than 90% of patients with eating disorders are female, and more than 75% are adolescents when they first develop their disorder (6). More than 95% of the patients are Caucasian, but the prevalence of eating disorders among Hispanic, Native American, Black, and Asian-American females is considerably higher than previously suspected (7).

The etiology of eating disorders is unknown. Sociocultural, psychodevelopmental, genetic, and neurochemical factors contribute to the likelihood of being diagnosed with an eating disorder (5). Personal dissatisfaction with their appearance begins for many patients before and during puberty (8). One national survey revealed that 52% of girls aged 12–16 years in the United States perceived themselves as fat even though they were, in fact, normal weight (9). The age individuals begin to diet is decreasing. Research studies of 9–12 year olds have found that 75% admit to dieting in a given year (4). Another report shows that adolescent girls who are victims of physical or sexual violence have triple the risk for signs of eating disorders (10). In 2001, 7.8% of adolescent girls reported that they took laxatives or vomited for weight control (11). Patients with an eating disorder may manifest in various presentations that gynecologists may see in their clinical practice (see Box 5). The American College of Obstetricians and Gynecologists recommends that all adolescents should be screened annually for eating disorders. Particularly, young women seeking gynecologic care

Once limited to the affluent upper class, eating disorders no longer recognize socioeconomic, racial, and ethnic barriers ...

require screening for eating disorders when they present with a history of amenorrhea for more than three cycles or abnormal menses; refusal to maintain body weight at or above a normal weight for age and height; recurrent dieting when not overweight; use of self-induced vomiting, laxatives, starvation, or diuretics to lose weight; distorted body image; body mass index (BMI) below the 5th percentile; excessive exercising; or the characteristic findings indicative of an eating disorder on physical or gynecologic examination (12). Two additional symptoms patients with eating disorders may present with are vague abdominal discomfort associated with constipation or depressed mood. (See "Primary and Preventive Health Care for Female Adolescents" chapter for more on periodic screening for adolescent patients.)

Once an eating disorder has been identified, it is important to inquire about suicidal ideation because eating disorders are associated with suicide as a result of mood disorders (13). To deal with these issues in a timely manner, it is advised to know the community resources. Medical and mental health consultants willing to accept patients into treatment should be identified once the conditions are recognized. Eating disorder consultants or multidisciplinary clinics may provide optimal care.

Anorexia Nervosa

Definition

The diagnostic criteria for anorexia includes (14): 1) refusal to maintain body weight at or above a minimally normal weight for age and height (eg, weight loss leading to maintenance of body weight less than 85% of normal weight for age and height or failure to make recommended weight gain during periods of growth, leading to body weight less than 85% of that expected); 2) intense fear of gaining weight or becoming fat, even though underweight; 3) disturbance in the way the body weight or shape is experienced, undue influence of body weight or shape on self-image, or denial of the seriousness of the current low body weight; and 4) amenorrhea in postmenarchal females. See Box 6 for definitions of the two subtypes of anorexia.

History and Physical Examination

Medical assessment of anorexia focuses on the history of the behavior (ie, its onset, duration, associated symptoms, and signs). Patients will frequently report amenorrhea before actual weight loss in up to 20% of reported

---

Box 5. Common Presentations of Eating Disorders

Gynecologic presentations
- Amenorrhea
- Menstrual irregularity
- Constipation or abdominal pain
- Sexually transmitted disease
- Contraceptive needs
- Pelvic pain
- Atrophic vaginitis
- Breast atrophy

Other presentations
- Depression
- Weakness
- Sports injuries and fractures
- Mouth sores
- Pharyngeal trauma
- Dental caries
- Heartburn
- Chest pain
- Muscle cramps
- Bloody diarrhea
- Bleeding or easy bruising
- Fainting
- Routine medical care

cases (4). The patient should be questioned about her weight (maximum, minimum, and ideal), menstrual history and pattern, satisfaction with how she looks (body image), exercise regimen, current and past medication, eating habits, diet history, binge or purge behaviors, laxative or diet pill use, sexual history, substance abuse, suicidal ideation, and symptoms of depression (13).

The physical examination begins with vital signs and height and weight measurements. If anorexia is suspected, the patient should be weighed wearing only a hospital gown with all clothing removed. The patient's height, bone structure, and BMI determine the appropriateness of the weight. If her BMI is below the 5th percentile, an assessment should be made to determine the possibility of anorexia. Findings on physical examination typical of anorexia may include low body temperature, bradycardia, orthostatic hypotension, dry skin with lanugo hair, acrocyanosis, mitral valve prolapse, scaphoid abdomen with retained stool, ankle and leg edema, and the absence of fat pads over the scapulae (13). Gynecologic examination, when indicated, may demonstrate the consequences of reduced estrogen (eg, pubertal delay, atrophic vaginitis, and breast atrophy). Pregnancy testing and sexually transmitted disease (STD) screening should be obtained in sexually active patients, if indicated. Differential diagnosis includes new onset diabetes, adrenal insufficiency, primary depression, schizophrenia, inflammatory bowel disease, and abdominal masses and central nervous system lesions that may cause vomiting. Initial office laboratory studies include complete blood count, urinalysis, electrolytes, glucose, thyroid screening, phosphorous, magnesium, and erythrocyte sedimentation rate (13, 15). Baseline follicle-stimulating hormone and luteinizing hormone levels also should be obtained.

TREATMENT

It is important to assess the need for emergency admission of the patient who has anorexia to the hospital because life-threatening conditions may arise (see Box 7). A team approach is recommended to treat a patient with anorexia and other eating disorders. The treatment team consists of a medical provider, a mental health therapist, and a nutritionist or dietitian. In an adolescent, a family therapist is recommended to help family members deal with the illness. Some patients prefer working in a group therapy setting. Treatment can be either outpatient or inpatient (see Box 8). It can take sev-

---

Box 6. Subtypes of Anorexia

Binge-eating/purging—An individual who is regularly engaged in binge-eating or purging (or both) behavior through self-induced vomiting or the misuse of laxatives, diuretics, or enemas during the current episode of anorexia nervosa.

Restricting—An individual who is not engaged in binge-eating or purging behavior during the current episode of anorexia nervosa. Weight loss is accomplished through dieting, fasting, or excessive exercise.

Some patients engage in cycles of binge eating and purging in addition to frequent fasting.

Reprinted and adapted with permission from the Diagnostic and Statistical Manual of Mental Disorders, Fourth Edition, Text Revision. Copyright 2000 American Psychiatric Association.

eral years to guide the patient to resolution of her eating disorder (15). Different medications have been used over the years. Although there are no studies that prove selective serotonin reuptake inhibitors (SSRIs) make a causal difference in the outcome of the illness, many patients show improvement in their depressive symptoms.

Long-term recovery is dependent on the individual patient. In one study that followed patients with anorexia for 10–15 years, 76% of the patients experienced full recovery, 10% experienced partial recovery, and 14% failed to achieve any recovery (16).

HEALTH CONSEQUENCES

The consequences of malnutrition in the patient with anorexia are determined by the severity of the starvation and its duration. The annual mortality rate associated with anorexia is more than 12 times the death rate in the general population of young women (17).

The impact of anorexia on skeletal health is significant. Patients with anorexia have a bone mineral density 25% lower than age-matched controls (18). Unfortunately, the density of trabecular bone (spine and femoral neck) may remain low even after recovery to a normal weight (19). Amenorrhea in an adolescent with anorexia of as short a period as a few months may be associated with osteopenia and, later on, osteoporosis (18).

Box 7. Criteria for Inpatient Treatment Program*

- Severe malnutrition (weight <75% expected body weight)
- Dehydration
- Electrolyte disturbance
- Cardiac dysrhythmia
- Physiologic instability (eg, severe bradycardia, hypotension, hypothermia, orthostatic changes)
- Arrested growth and development
- Failure of outpatient treatment
- Acute food refusal
- Uncontrollable binge eating and purging
- Acute medical complications of malnutrition, such as syncope, seizures, and cardiac failure
- Acute psychiatric emergencies, such as suicidal ideation or acute psychosis, and any co-morbid diagnosis that interferes with treatment, such as severe depression, obsessive–compulsive disorder, or severe family dysfunction

*Any of these symptoms and behaviors would justify hospitalization.
Adapted from Fisher M, Golden NH, Katzman DK, Kreipe RE, Rees J, Schebendach J, et al. Eating disorders in adolescents: a background paper. J Adolesc Health 1995;16: 420–37.

Bulimia Nervosa

DEFINITION

The word bulimia means hunger of an "ox." Patients with bulimia consume large amounts of food, frequently in secret, and then participate in inappropriate behaviors, such as purging, fasting, or excessive fasting to compensate for the volume consumed. Patients with purging bulimia frequently resort to laxatives and diuretics in a further attempt to reduce the effect of the caloric overload. Unlike patients with anorexia who feel elated with control of their intake, patients with bulimia feel lack of control over the amount and type of food eaten and experience feelings of guilt

Box 8. Treatment for Eating Disorders

In the absence of special training and experience in the management of eating disorders, the obstetrician–gynecologist is well advised to refer the patient for specialized care once an eating disorder is diagnosed or strongly suspected.

Outpatient

- A team approach is recommended for the outpatient treatment of all types of eating disorders.
- The treatment team can include the health care provider, individual therapist, nutritionist, and family therapist for the younger adolescent. In most cases, an obstetrician–gynecologist would not have the expertise to lead the team, but could still be an important part of the team.
- The team should communicate regularly on the patient's progress.
- Treatment goals should be identified and negotiated with the patient.
- The criteria for medical or psychiatric admission should be clearly identified for the patient and her family. Medical admission usually is based on the failure to comply with the meal plan resulting in further weight loss and a deterioration of vital signs.

Inpatient

- Inpatient treatment is required when weight loss has been prolonged and life-threatening conditions develop (see Box 7).
- Treatment emphasis should be placed on both the physical and psychologic needs of the patient.
- Many inpatient programs also have a step-down day program, which allows a gradual reentry of the patient into a healthy lifestyle. These day programs provide the additional support needed around meal times.

Pharmacology

- To date, there are no long-term studies specifically identifying a medication that treats eating disorders.
- The serotonin reuptake class of drugs has shown to have some benefit in the short term (first 2 months) for decreasing the number of binge episodes. They also have proved helpful in treating the depression and obsessive–compulsive ideation frequently seen in patients with eating disorders.* They should not be relied on as the sole or primary treatment.
- Estrogen and progestin replacement is advocated after 1 year of amenorrhea in girls with eating disorders. Studies have not confirmed a benefit of this therapy in treating osteopenia except in patients with less than 70% ideal body weight.† However, there are other secondary gains to normalizing the hormone levels (improved sense of well-being, improved muscle strength, reduced sleep disturbance, increased libido, and reduced likelihood of night sweats).
- For the severely restrictive patient, multivitamin and calcium supplements are advised.
- A stool softener also is recommended for patients with anorexia because they often are constipated because of decreased gut mobility caused by starvation.

---

*Kreipe RE, Dukarm CP. Eating disorders in adolescents and older children. Pediatr Rev 1999;20:410–21.

†Klibanski A, Biller BM, Schoenfeld DA, Herzog DB, Saxe VC. The effects of estrogen administration on trabecular bone loss in young women with anorexia nervosa. J Clin Endocrinol Metab 1995;80:898–904.

over their inability to stop the binge eating and purging (14). Another significant psychologic difference between patients with anorexia and patients with bulimia is asking for help. Patients with bulimia often are disgusted with their behavior and want help in stopping it, while patients with anorexia identify with their eating disorder and resist treatment efforts (13).

History and Physical Examination

Patients with bulimia are not easily recognized. Their weight is typically normal to slightly overweight (within 10–20% of the expected standard). Because the physical findings can be subtle, unlike the obvious weight loss of patients with anorexia, eating behaviors, such as a history of vomiting or use of laxatives or diuretics to control weight, should be included in the review of systems during routine health care. Bulimia should be considered in patients with polycystic ovary syndrome (20).

The physical examination of the patient with bulimia is frequently normal. When signs and symptoms are present, they represent the consequences of vomiting and the abuse of laxatives or diuretics. Pelvic pain and constipation are related to a variety of factors including abnormal food intake and laxative use. Other typical findings include scalp hair loss (diffuse thinning), parotid swelling (secondary to vomiting), abnormal dentition with gum recession, gum disease, enamel erosion of the teeth, scars on fingers (Russell's sign), and perianal erythema (5, 13). Unlike patients with anorexia, patients with bulimia usually have menstrual cycles although they tend to be irregular. The laboratory evaluation of a patient with bulimia includes complete blood count with differential, electrolytes, blood urea nitrogen and creatinine, glucose, calcium, phosphorous, and magnesium concentrations (13).

Bulimia often is associated with impulsive, risk-taking behavior that can lead to STDs and unintended pregnancy (15, 21, 22). Careful sexual history taking may be advisable for patients with bulimia as well as obtaining an eating history for adolescents with STDs.

Treatment

It is important to determine if the patient who has bulimia needs to be admitted immediately to the hospital because life-threatening conditions may arise (see Box 7). Treatment involves a team approach—medical supervision, psychologic therapy, and nutritional counseling. It can include inpatient or outpatient care (see Box 8). The prognosis remains guarded because of the habituation and ease of performing the behavior.

Health Consequences

Purging may be life threatening. Hypokalemia and hypophosphatemia are potentially lethal. Resultant gastrointestinal disorders include pancreatitis, esophagitis and esophageal rupture, Mallory-Weiss lesions, paralytic ileus secondary to laxative abuse, and cathartic colon. Hypomagnesemia results in muscle cramps, weakness, and restlessness. Pulmonary complications of aspiration pneumonia and pneumomediastinum can result from vomiting. Irreversible cardiomyopathy may occur in patients with bulimia who use ipecac to induce vomiting (23).

Binge Eating Disorder

Definition

Binge eating disorder is a variant of bulimia. The patient with binge eating disorder also consumes large quantities of food, but does not purge or engage in compensatory behaviors, such as excessive exercise or prolonged fasting. Binge eaters may eat regular meals and snacks throughout the day. Research has shown that dieting (fasting), chronic restrained eating, and excessive exercise may be important triggers for binge eating disorder (6).

History and Physical Examination

Physicians should consider binge eating disorder in every obese patient with polycystic ovary syndrome (20). Identifying the patient with binge eating disorder requires a history sensitive to the issue of binge eating. The patient with binge eating disorder often has an associated psychologic diagnosis, most commonly depression.

Obese binge eating disorder patients have the laboratory profile typical of the morbidly obese. Morbid obesity is more commonly associated with binge eating disorder than with bulimia. The fasting insulin level is elevated. The serum glucose level also may be abnormally high if type 2 diabetes has developed. The cholesterol, high-density lipoprotein and low-density lipoprotein cholesterol, and triglyceride levels may be abnormal. Liver function tests will be abnormal and reflect fatty degeneration of the liver when present. For the normal weight binge eating disorder patient, the body's compensatory mechanisms would normalize the laboratory values.

Treatment

Research on the etiology of binge eating disorder suggests that treatment should focus on healthy weight-control techniques, not accepting the media's sociocultural pressures to be thin, eliminating the thin ideal of beauty, and improving the self-esteem of young adolescent women. There has been case-based evidence that SSRI's decrease the number of binge episodes and may help prevent relapse among patients in remission, although the SSRI's mechanism of action for treatment of this disorder has not been identified (6). Long-term studies are not available.

Health Consequences

Binge eating disorder has a persistent course and often is associated with co-morbid psychopathology (depression), which contributes to medical complications. Because patients with binge eating disorder are not purging, they do not have the risks associated with vomiting and the use of laxatives and diuretics. Massive caloric intake often results in obesity with its attendant complications.

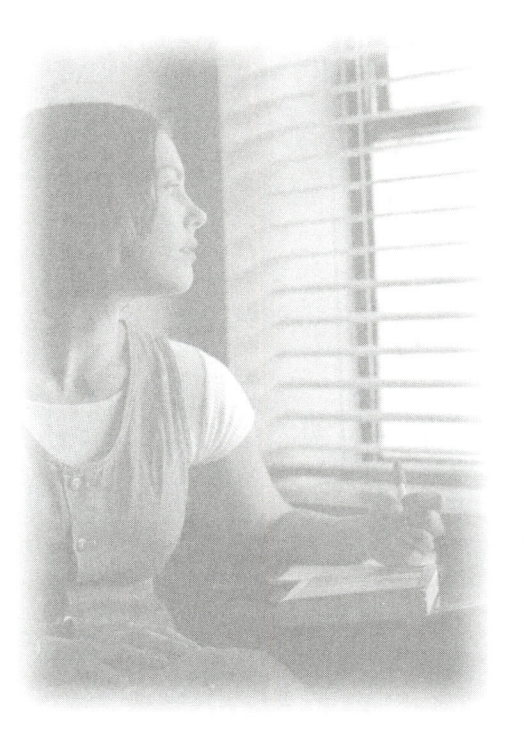

Female Athlete Triad

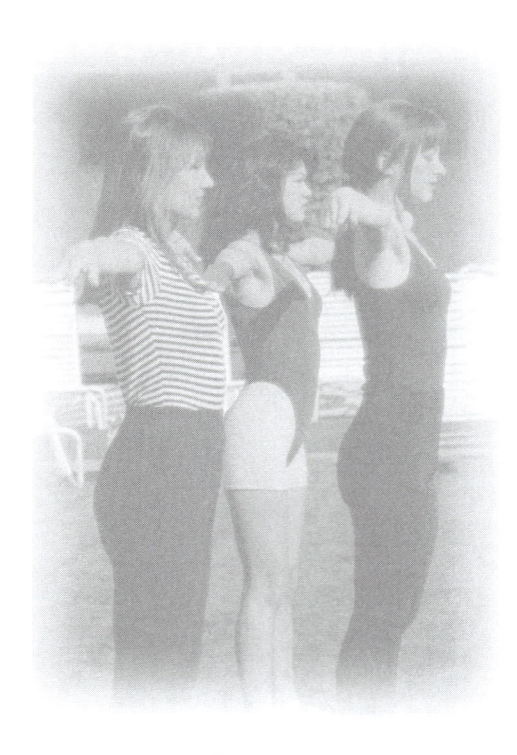

Definition

In 1992, the American College of Sports Medicine coined the term "female athlete triad," which refers to the inter-relatedness of disordered eating, amenorrhea, and osteoporosis that are associated with athletic training (24). The disordered eating ranges from severe restricting and purging to obsessive avoidance of fat and chemical preservatives. Although the exact prevalence of female athlete triad is unknown, the prevalence of disordered eating in female college athletes varies from 15% to 62% (24). The athletes most at risk for developing the triad are those in whom a low body weight and lean physique are desired (eg, gymnast, figure skater, ballet dancer, and runner) (24).

History and Physical Examination

Excessive physical training before puberty may delay menarche. Amenorrhea in athletes is the absence of three or more consecutive menstrual cycles in the postpubertal female. Pregnancy must be ruled out. Oligomenorrhea is a common finding in female athletes. Premature bone loss and inadequate bone formation characterizes osteoporosis in the athlete. These young women experience a reduction in bone mass, deterioration of bone microarchitecture, and a fragile skeleton, which results in an increased risk of fractures.

Treatment

The management of the female athlete triad stresses healthy behaviors while supporting the young woman's interest in sports. Athletic participation and exercise are healthy. It is inappropriate to deny participation in sports because of the risk of developing the female athlete triad. Once female athlete triad is recognized, however, prompt intervention is advised. As with other eating disorders, proper nutrition is essential, including an adequate intake of calcium (1,300 mg daily). Studies have supported a positive relationship between calcium intake and normal bone density (25, 26).

Health Consequences

Exercise favors bone formation, with weight-bearing exercise being the most effective. However, when excessive exercise leads to amenorrhea, the benefits are lost. Normal estrogen levels are essential in maintaining normal bone density, and amenorrhea associated with a low estrogen level results in low bone mineral density (27). Bone demineralization in the too thin patient with anorexia is rapid, often measurable within 1 year of onset with weight loss and amenorrhea (28). Studies clearly demonstrate that athletes with regular menstrual cycles have higher bone density than their counterparts with amenorrhea (27, 29).

The incidence of premature osteoporosis is unknown. An increased risk of stress fractures and scoliosis has been reported in ballet dancers with delayed menarche and prolonged intervals of amenorrhea (30). Female athlete triad disorders can decrease physical performance and cause morbidity and mortality. Further research is needed to identify its causes, prevalence, and consequences.

Prevention of Eating Disorders

Because the definitive etiology of eating disorders is unknown, prevention remains a mystery. A familial tendency has been noted as well as characteristic personality traits, such as perfectionism, low self-esteem, and need for control (4). In general, emphasizing a healthy lifestyle, avoiding extremes, and reinforcing the acceptance of all body types will provide young women with a positive environment. Gynecologists can play a vital role in promoting young women's health. They have the opportunity to provide the structured guidance to counteract society's unrealistic expectations that equate extreme thinness with beauty and to work with local, state, and national initiatives to prevent eating disorders.

References

1. Becker AE, Grinspoon SK, Klibanski A, Herzog DB. Eating disorders. N Engl J Med 1999;340:1092–8.
2. Fisher M, Golden NH, Katzman DK, Kreipe RE, Rees J, Schebendach J, et al. Eating disorders in adolescents: a background paper. J Adolesc Health 1995;16:420–37.
3. Lucas AR, Beard CM, O'Fallon WM, Kurland LT. 50-year trends in the incidence of anorexia nervosa in Rochester, Minn.: a population-based study. Am J Psychiatry 1991;148:917–22.
4. Rosen DS. Eating disorders. Female Pat 1995;20(10):12–4, 16–8.
5. Yates A. Current perspectives on the eating disorders: I. History, psychological and biological aspects. J Am Acad Child Adolesc Psychiatry 1989;28: 813–28.
6. Kreipe RE, Dukarm CP. Eating disorders in adolescents and older children. Pediatr Rev 1999;20:410–21.
7. Crago M, Shisslak CM, Estes LS. Eating disturbances among American minority groups: a review. Int J Eat Disord 1996;19:239–48.
8. Chaum E, Herzog DB. New directions in anorexia nervosa and bulimia nervosa. Curr Opin Pediatr 1990;2:641–7.
9. Strauss RS. Self-reported weight status and dieting in a cross-sectional sample of young adolescents: National Health and Nutrition Examination Survey III. Arch Pediatr Adolesc Med 1999;153:741–7.
10. Schoen C, Davis K, Collins KS, Greenberg L, Des Roches C, Abrams M. The Commonwealth Fund Survey of the health of adolescent girls. New York: The Commonwealth Fund; 1997.
11. Grunbaum JA, Kann L, Kinchen SA, Williams B, Ross JG, Lowry R, et al. Youth risk behavior surveillance—United States, 2001. MMWR Surveill Summ 2002;51(4):1–62.

12. American College of Obstetricians and Gynecologists. Guidelines for women's health care. 2nd ed. Washington, DC: ACOG; 2002.
13. Davis AJ, Grace E. Dying to be thin: patients with anorexia and bulimia. A continuing education monograph. Raritan (NJ): Ortho-McNeil Pharmaceutical; 1999.
14. American Psychiatric Association. Diagnostic and statistical manual of mental disorders: DSM-IV-TR. 4th ed., text revision. Washington, DC: APA; 2000.
15. Kreipe RE, Mou SM. Eating disorders in adolescents and young adults. Obstet Gynecol Clin North Am 2000;27:101–24.
16. Strober M, Freeman R, Morrell W. The long-term course of severe anorexia nervosa in adolescents: survival analysis of recovery, relapse, and outcome predictors over 10–15 years in a prospective study. Int J Eat Disord 1997;22: 339–60.
17. Sullivan PF. Mortality in anorexia nervosa. Am J Psychiatry 1995;152: 1073–4.
18. Bachrach LK, Guido D, Katzman D, Litt IF, Marcus R. Decreased bone density in adolescent girls with anorexia nervosa. Pediatrics 1990;86;440–7.
19. Klibanski A, Biller BM, Schoenfeld DA, Herzog DB, Saxe VC. The effects of estrogen administration on trabecular bone loss in young women with anorexia nervosa. J Clin Endocrinol Metab 1995;80:898–904.
20. McCluskey S, Evans C, Lacey JH, Pearce JM, Jacobs H. Polycystic ovary syndrome and bulimia. Fertil Steril 1991;55:287–91.
21. Practice guideline for the treatment of patients with eating disorders (revision). American Psychiatric Association Work Group on Eating Disorders. Am J Psychiatry 2000;157(suppl):1–39.
22. Lacey JH. Bulimia nervosa, binge eating, and psychogenic vomiting: a controlled treatment study and long term outcome. Br Med J (Clin Res Ed) 1983;286:1609–13.
23. Mitchell JE, Pomeroy C, Adson DE. Managing medical complications. In: Garner DM, Garfinkel PE, editors. Handbook of treatment for eating disorders. 2nd ed. New York: Guilford Press; 1997. p. 383–93.
24. Hobart JA, Smucker DR. The female athlete triad. Am Fam Physician 2000; 61:3357–64, 3367.
25. Merrilees MJ, Smart EJ, Gilchrist NL, Frampton C, Turner JG, Hooke E, et al. Effects of diary food supplements on bone mineral density in teenage girls. Eur J Nutr 2000;39:256–62.
26. Moyer-Mileur L, Xie B, Ball S, Bainbridge C, Stadler D, Jee WS. Predictors of bone mass by peripheral quantitative computed tomography in early adolescent girls. J Clin Densitom 2001;4:313–23.
27. Myburgh KH, Bachrach LK, Lewis B, Kent K, Marcus R. Low bone mineral density at axial and appendicular sites in amenorrheic athletes. Med Sci Sports Exerc 1993;25:1197–202.
28. Powers PS. Osteoporosis and eating disorders. J Pediatr Adolesc Gynecol 1999;12:51–7.
29. Gibson JH, Harries M, Mitchell A, Godfrey R, Lunt M, Reeve J. Determinants of bone density and prevalence of osteopenia among female runners in their second to seventh decades of age. Bone 2000;26:591–8.
30. Warren MP, Brooks-Gunn J, Hamilton LH, Warren LF, Hamilton WG. Scoliosis and fractures in young ballet dancers. Relation to delayed menarche and secondary amenorrhea. N Engl J Med 1986;314:1348–53.

Resources

ACOG Resources

American College of Obstetricians and Gynecologists. Eating disorders. ACOG Patient Education Pamphlet AP144. Washington, DC: ACOG; 2000.

American College of Obstetricians and Gynecologists. Tool kit for teen care. Washington, DC: ACOG; 2003.

American College of Obstetricians and Gynecologists. Weight control: eating right and keeping fit. ACOG Patient Education Pamphlet AP064. Washington, DC: ACOG; 1999.

Other Resources

The following lists are for information purposes only. Referral to these sources and web sites does not imply the endorsement of ACOG. These lists are not meant to be comprehensive. The exclusion of a source or web site does not reflect the quality of that source or web site. Please note that web sites are subject to change without notice.

Academy for Eating Disorders
6728 Old McLean Village Drive
McLean, VA 22101-3906
Tel: (703) 556-9222
Fax: (703) 556-8729
Web: www.aedweb.org

American Academy of Family Physicians
11400 Tomahawk Creek Parkway
Leawood, KS 66211-2672
Tel: (913) 906-6000
Web: www.aafp.org

American Academy of Pediatrics
141 Northwest Point Boulevard
Elk Grove Village, IL 60007-1098
Tel: (847) 228-5005
Fax: (847) 228-5097
Web: www.aap.org

American Anorexia Bulimia Association, Inc
165 W 46th Street, Suite 1108
New York, NY 10036
Tel: (212) 575-6200
Web: www.aabainc.org
E-mail: amanbu@aol.com

American Dietetic Association
216 West Jackson Boulevard
Chicago, IL 60606-6995
Tel: (312) 899-0040
Fax: (312) 899-1979
Web: www.eatright.org

American Psychiatric Association
1400 K Street NW
Washington, DC 20005
Tel: 888-357-7924
Fax: (202) 682-6850
Web: www.psych.org/

American Psychological Association
750 First Street NE
Washington, DC 20002-4242
Tel: 800-374-2721; (202) 336-5510
Web: www.apa.org

Anorexia Nervosa and Related Eating Disorders, Inc.
PO Box 5102
Eugene, OR 97405
Tel: (541) 344-1144
Web: www.anred.com

National Association of Anorexia and Associated Disorders
PO Box 7
Highland Park, IL 60035
Tel: (847) 831-3438
Fax: (847) 433-4632
Web: www.anad.org

Society for Adolescent Medicine
1916 NW Copper Oaks Circle
Blue Springs, MO 64015
Tel: (816) 224-8010
Web: www.adolescenthealth.org

Resources for Your Patients

Go Ask Alice! (by Columbia University Health Education Program)
Lerner Hall
2920 Broadway, 7th Floor
MC 2608
New York, NY 10027
Tel: (212) 854-5453
Fax: (212) 854-8949
Web: www.goaskalice.columbia.edu

Center for Young Women's Health
Children's Hospital
333 Longwood Avenue, 5th floor
Boston, MA 02115
Tel: (617) 355-CYWH (2994)
Fax: (617) 232-3136
Web: www.youngwomenshealth.org

National Eating Disorders Association
603 Stewart Street, Suite 803
Seattle, WA 98101
Tel: (206) 382-3587
Web: www.nationaleatingdisorders.org/

National Women's Health Information Center (by DHHS Office on Women's Health)
8550 Arlington Boulevard, Suite 300
Fairfax, VA 22031
Tel: 800-994-WOMAN
Web: www.4woman.org; www.4girls.gov

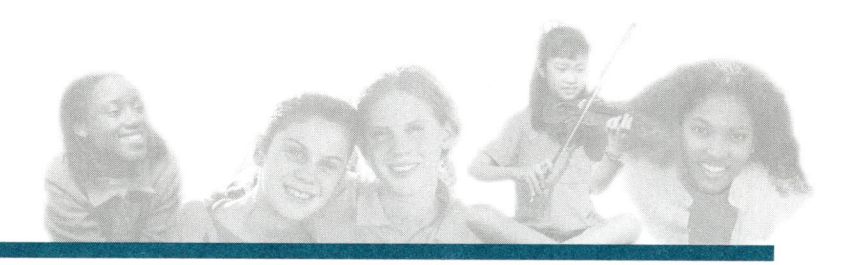

Preventing Adolescent Suicide

Key points

➢ Suicide is the third leading cause of death in adolescents (aged 15–24 years). Suicide among younger adolescents (aged 10–14 years) is rare but increasing.

➢ Female adolescents attempt suicide nearly twice as frequently as male adolescents, although male adolescents have higher completion rates.

➢ The majority of all adolescent suicides are committed by whites, but suicide rates are significantly higher than national rates among Native Americans, and increasing rapidly among blacks.

➢ Firearms are the most commonly used method for completed suicides both among male and female adolescents. Poisoning (including drug overdose) is a common method among female adolescents, and is thought to be the most frequent method of attempted suicide.

➢ Risk factors for suicide and suicide attempt include presence of mental disorder; family history of psychiatric disorder; substance abuse; previous suicide attempt; certain physical disorders that cause functional impairment; history of sexual or physical abuse; easy access to lethal weapons; living in a nontraditional setting; being gay, lesbian or bisexual; stressful life events; being pregnant or parenting; being divorced; and exposure to a recent suicide or suicide attempt in a family, community or peer group, or through media coverage.

➢ All adolescents, especially pregnant or parenting adolescents, should be asked about a history of childhood sexual or physical abuse and evaluated for their risk for suicidal ideation and attempt.

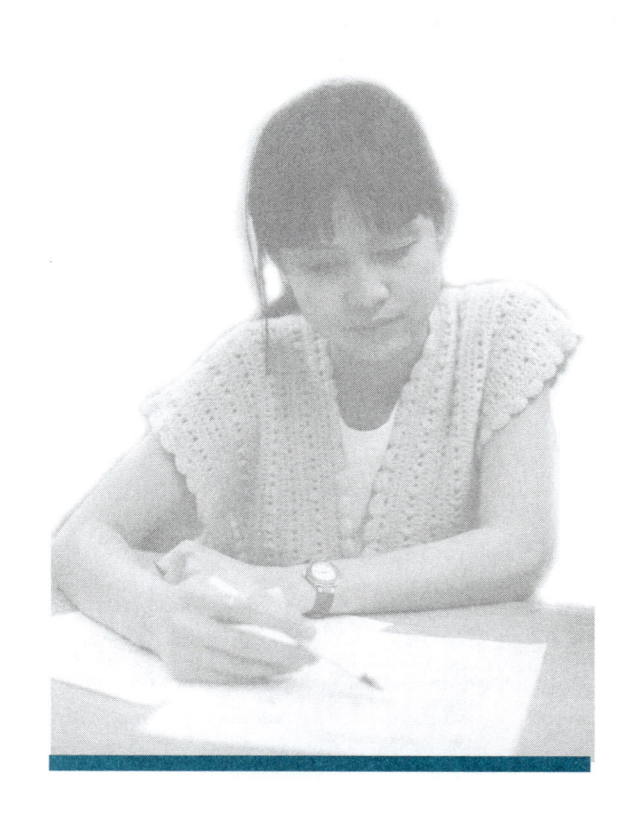

*E*very day in this country, 86 individuals take their own lives and another 1,500 attempt suicide, making it the eighth leading cause of death in the United States. (1). Recognizing that suicide is a serious public health problem, then U.S. Surgeon General David Satcher issued a National Strategy for Suicide Prevention on May 2001, laying out 11 goals designed to reduce and prevent this problem (2) (see Box 9). Suicide is not only a problem among adults; it is an even more serious problem among adolescents (see Box 10). The rate of adolescent suicide in the United States tripled between 1952 and 1992, although it decreased slightly in the late 1990s (3, 4). After accidents and homicide, suicide is the third leading cause of death in those aged 15–24 years and accounts for 12.8% (3,994) of all deaths in this group (5). Suicide is rare in children and younger adolescents, but it is increasing rapidly. Between 1980 and 1997, the suicide rate among individuals aged 15–19 years increased by 11%; among those aged 10–14 years, it increased by 109% (6). There are estimated to be 50–100 suicide attempts for every completed suicide among adolescents (7, 8). Nineteen percent of students in grades 9–12 reported having seriously considered attempting suicide in the past year, and 14.8% reported having made a specific plan to attempt suicide (9).

Although suicide rates among adolescent males exceed rates for females by nearly five to one (5), females attempt suicide more frequently (9). Approximately 11% of female students in grades 9–12 reported having attempted suicide compared with 6.2% of males. Overall, Hispanic female students (15.9%) were more likely than white and black female students (10.3% and 9.8%, respectively) to have attempted suicide (9).

White males and females account for the majority of all adolescent suicides. However, the suicide rate among Native-American adolescents aged 15–24 years ranged from 2.4 to 2.8 times higher than the national rate (10). The suicide rate is increasing rapidly among black adolescents; the rate for black adolescents aged 15–19 years increased 126% between 1980 and 1995, compared with 19% for white adolescents (11).

Nineteen percent of students in grades 9–12 reported having seriously considered attempting suicide in the past year...

Methods of Suicide

The three most common methods of completed suicide among all adolescents aged 15–24 years are by 1) firearms, 2) suffocation (including hanging), and 3) poisoning (including drug overdose) (12). Although firearms are more commonly used by adolescent males and contribute to their higher rate of completed suicides, most adolescent females who complete suicide also do so with a firearm. Poisoning, as a method of completed suicide, is more common among female adolescents than males (12), and it is thought to be the most frequent method of attempted suicides. The lethality of attempted suicide is increasing because of a corresponding increase in the use of firearms by suicidal adolescents. Between 1980 and 1997, firearms accounted for 62% of the increase in overall suicide rates for 15–19 year olds (6); in 1999, they accounted for 59.3% of suicides among individuals aged 15–24 years (5). One factor that may explain the prominent role of firearms in adolescent suicide is the high rate of gun ownership. Thirty-five percent of U.S. households now contain a gun (13), and studies have shown that adolescents who commit suicide by firearms are significantly more likely to have a firearm in their home. (14)

Risk Factors

Risk factors for suicide or suicide attempts are listed in Box 11 (14–16). Also vulnerable are physically or sexually abused adolescents, delinquents, runaways, and any adolescent living in nontraditional settings, such as juvenile detention centers, prisons, halfway houses, or group homes (17). Adolescent girls who endure physical or sexual violence by dating partners are at higher risk of considering or attempting suicide than nonvictims (18). Because very high-achieving adolescents, who may have personalities of rigid perfectionism, and impulsive adolescents also are at increased risk of suicide, "problem teens" are not the only group that clinicians need to evaluate for suicide potential. Several studies have reported that gay, lesbian, and bisexual adolescents have higher rates for suicide thoughts and attempts than heterosexual adolescents, although there are no statistical data to report that completed suicide rates are higher among the gay, lesbian, and bisexual population (19, 20). Stressful life events, such as school difficulties or failure, legal difficulties, breakup of a relationship, and social isolation, often precede a suicide attempt (1, 21). It is important to recognize that stressors adults perceive as trivial may be very significant

---

Box 9. National Strategy for Suicide Prevention: Goals and Objectives for Action

1. Promote awareness that suicide is a public health problem that is preventable.
2. Develop broad-based support for suicide prevention.
3. Develop and implement strategies to reduce the stigma associated with being a consumer of mental health, substance abuse, and suicide prevention services.
4. Develop and implement suicide prevention programs.
5. Promote efforts to reduce access to lethal means and methods of self-harm.
6. Implement training for recognition of at-risk behavior and delivery of effective treatment.
7. Develop and promote effective clinical and professional practices.
8. Improve access to and community linkages with mental health and substance abuse services.
9. Improve reporting and portrayals of suicidal behavior, mental illness, and substance abuse in the entertainment and news media.
10. Promote and support research on suicide and suicide prevention.
11. Improve and expand surveillance systems.

U.S. Department of Health and Human Services. National strategy for suicide prevention: goals and objectives for action. Rockville (MD): USDHHS; 2001.

to adolescents, precipitating a threat to self-worth and suicidal behavior. Conflicts with parents and a lack of parent–child communication also may act as a risk factor (1, 21).

Although pregnancy itself may not be a risk factor among adolescent girls, several studies show that pregnant adolescent girls and adolescent mothers with a history of sexual or physical abuse are at three to seven times higher risk for suicide ideation and attempt than those without a history of abuse (22, 23). Also, divorced adolescent females are at increased risk for suicide. It has been suggested that women at all ages do not fully anticipate the economic and other hardships associated with divorce and are, thus, ill-prepared for the depression and role conflict that may follow the dissolution of their marriages (24).

Both fictional and nonfictional media coverage of suicide, such as intensive reporting of the suicide of a celebrity or the fictional representation of a suicide in a popular movie or TV show, can serve as a trigger for vulnerable adolescents to act on suicidal thoughts. Exposure to a recent suicide or suicide attempt in one's family, peer group, or community also can result in an increase in suicide in adolescents (1).

Depression is associated very strongly with suicide. The defining symptoms of depression are five or more of the following (including at least 1 of the first 2) nearly everyday, all day, and for at least 2 weeks: depressed mood; diminished interest or pleasure; weight loss when not dieting or weight gain; insomnia or hypersomnia; fatigue or loss of energy; psychomotor agitation or retardation; feeling of worthlessness or excessive or inappropriate guilt; indecisiveness or diminished ability to think or concentrate; and recurrent thoughts of death, suicidal ideation, suicide attempt, or plan (16). Depression in adolescents, however, may not have the same clinical manifestations as in adults and may present as (16):

- Somatic complaints
- Irritability
- Social withdrawal

Box 10. Epidemiology of Adolescent Suicide

- Suicide is the third leading cause of death in adolescents (aged 15–24 years).
- Suicide among younger adolescents (aged 10–14 years) is rare but increasing.
- Female adolescents attempt suicide twice as frequently as male adolescents, although male adolescents have higher completion rates.
- The majority of all adolescent suicides are committed by whites, but suicide rates are significantly high among Native Americans, and increasing rapidly among blacks.

Box 11. Risk Factors for Suicide or Suicide Attempts

- Presence of mental disorder
- Family history of psychiatric disorder
- Substance abuse
- Previous suicide attempt
- Certain physical disorders that cause functional impairment
- History of sexual or physical abuse
- Easy access to lethal weapons
- Living in nontraditional setting
- Being gay, lesbian, or bisexual
- Stressful life events
- Being a parent or pregnancy (especially those with history of abuse and those under stress)
- Divorce
- Exposure to a recent suicide or suicide attempt in a family, community, or friends, or through media coverage

Sexual acting-out also may be a symptom of depression and may cause the adolescent to come to the attention of the obstetrician–gynecologist. Although certain circumstances or events may seem to make depression more "understandable," they in no way decrease the importance of depression as a suicide risk factor.

Risk Assessment and Prevention

Obstetrician–gynecologists regularly come into contact with individuals at risk for suicide and have an opportunity for the primary prevention of adolescent suicide. Adolescents contemplating suicide rarely offer that information as a presenting complaint. Often, however, they feel relieved to have the subject broached. Accordingly, physicians should ask directly about suicidal thoughts or fantasies. Most nonsuicidal patients will recognize an inquiry as indicative of concern and will not be offended. This subject may be addressed as part of background questioning in the context of family, school, and relationships. Because depressive symptoms are prevalent among pregnant and parenting adolescents, particularly those under stress and those without emotional and material support (25), physicians should assess their patients' risk for suicide once every trimester and at the postpartum visit. They also should ask all adolescent patients, especially pregnant and parenting adolescents, about a history of childhood sexual and physical abuse and evaluate their risk for suicide ideation and attempt. Questions should be asked in a nonjudgmental, direct, and nonthreatening manner: "Sometimes patients I've seen dealing with similar issues or problems get very down and start to question life itself. Does this happen to you?" If the answer is positive, it should be followed up with questions such as:

1. "Have you ever thought about suicide?"
2. "Are you thinking about suicide now?"
3. "Do you have a plan for committing suicide?" If yes, "What is your plan for committing suicide?"
4. "Have you ever attempted suicide?"

A positive response indicates the need for further questioning and an assessment of risk factors that could increase the suicide potential, such as easy access to a lethal weapon.

The degree of risk at any particular encounter should, to the extent possible, be fully assessed, and any response or intervention should be based on the level of risk. Significant insight is gained into the intent of the suicidal thought by analyzing the method and location of a planned suicide. Ingesting over-the-counter drugs in a location where the individual is likely to be discovered suggests a gesture that is looking for a response, whereas planning to use a firearm indicates strong intent on the part of the individual to accomplish the suicide (17, 26, 27).

Sexual acting-out also may be a symptom of depression and may cause the adolescent to come to the attention of the obstetrician–gynecologist.

Low Risk

A low-risk profile is one where there is ambivalence about wanting to die, no history of prior attempts, no alcohol or drug abuse, and no suicide plan. Additionally, this adolescent will have good family or peer support, will experience suicidal thoughts that are mild and transient, and will exhibit receptivity to getting help. This patient should be encouraged to enlist the assistance of family and significant others, consider counseling, and see a health professional weekly until the crisis is resolved.

Moderate Risk

A moderate-risk situation is one in which there is a psychiatric history or a history of suicide attempts. Use of drugs or alcohol may increase the risk of suicide. These patients may have more persistent thoughts of death or suicide, but their plans are only vaguely formulated or incompatible with the methods available to them. Involvement of families and mental health practitioners is critical. Although this situation calls for expedient linkage with a mental health professional, other health professionals can assist in this process. If depression is diagnosed and antidepressants are considered, referral to a psychiatrist or a provider with additional training may be appropriate.

High Risk

Evidence of high risk for suicide can include psychotic thinking, depression, or unremitting crisis, particularly when an adolescent has formulated a clear suicide plan and has the means to carry it out (such as a household firearm the patient intends to use) or when the ability to regulate behavior is compromised (eg, by substance use). Risk is especially high when the adolescent is cut off from or rejects resources or family support. If an adolescent appears to be at high risk for suicide, immediate referral to a mental health provider for surveillance, psychiatric evaluation, and psychotherapeutic intervention is indicated. If psychiatric evaluation is not immediately available, referral to a hospital emergency department for possible admission to protect the patient from self-harm may be indicated.

Conclusion

Counseling techniques for the suicidal adolescent should emphasize that the patient's current emotional state is temporary and treatable, offering alternatives to deal with the problem (26, 27). "No-suicide" contracts in which the adolescent pledges not to attempt suicide often are helpful but should not be relied on to prevent a suicide (28). Adolescents frequently request that their suicidal thoughts not be revealed. It is important to avoid being sworn to secrecy or making promises that cannot be kept because suicidal intent is not information that can be kept confidential. Moreover, it is imperative that, where applicable, the family of an adolescent at risk be advised immediately to make firearms in the home inaccessible and to lock up all medications kept anywhere in the home.

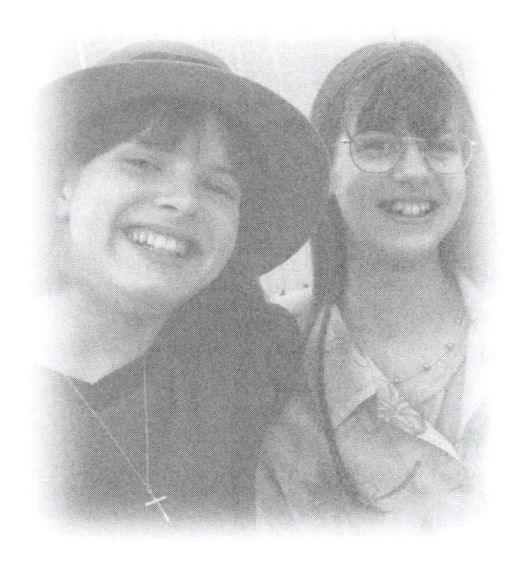

Physicians have an important role in addressing the problem of adolescent suicide. The increasing rate of adolescent suicide mandates an increasing awareness of depressive disorders, anxiety disorders, and chemical dependence in this population. Physicians should be prepared to assess suicide risk and, when necessary, provide immediate counseling or referral to mental health providers. Each patient encounter may be the only opportunity for intervention and may, in fact, be life saving.

References

1. U.S. Department of Health and Human Services. Mental health: a report of the Surgeon General. Rockville (MD): USDHHS; 1999.
2. National strategy for suicide prevention: goals and objectives for action. Rockville, Maryland: U.S. Department of Health and Human Services, Public Health Service, 2001. Available at http://www.mentalhealth.org/publications/allpubs/SMA01-3517/SMA01-3517.pdf. Retrieved October 17, 2002.
3. American Association of Suicidology. U.S.A. suicide: 1998 official final data. Washington, DC: AAS; 2001. Available at http://www.iusb.edu/~jmcintos/USA98Summary.htm. Retrieved October 17, 2002.
4. Suicide among children, adolescents, and young adults—United States, 1980–1992. MMWR Morb Mortal Wkly Rep 1995;44:289–91.
5. Anderson RN. Deaths: leading causes for 2000. Natl Vital Stat Rep 2002; 50(16):1–85.
6. National Center for Injury Prevention and Control. Suicide in the United States. Atlanta (GA): NCIPC; 2002. Available at http://www.cdc.gov/ncipc/factsheets/suifacts.htm. Retrieved October 17, 2002.
7. Gardner P, Hudson BL. Advance report of final mortality statistics, 1993. Monthly Vital Statistics Report; vol 44, no. 7 (suppl). Hyattsville (MD): National Center for Health Statistics, 1996.
8. Bearinger LH, Blum RW. Adolescent health. In: Wallace HM, Nelson RP, Sweeney PJ, editors. Maternal and child health practices. 4th ed. Oakland (CA): Third Party Publishing Company; 1994. p. 573–84.
9. Grunbaum JA, Kann L, Kinchen SA, Williams B, Ross JG, Lowry R, et al. Youth risk behavior surveillance—United States, 2001. MMWR Surveill Summ 2002;51(4):1–62.
10. Indian Health Service. Trends in Indian health, 1998-99. Rockville (MD): IHS, 2001.
11. Suicide among black youths—United States, 1980–1995. MMWR Morb Mortal Wkly Rep 1998;47:193–6.
12. National Center for Injury Prevention and Control. Leading causes of death reports. Atlanta (GA): NCIPC. Available at http://webapp.cdc.gov/sasweb/ncipc/leadcaus.html. Retrieved October 17, 2002.
13. Smith TW. 2001 National gun policy survey of the National Opinion Research Center: research findings. Chicago (IL): National Opinion Research Center; 2001.

14. Shah S, Hoffman RE, Wake L, Marine WM. Adolescent suicide and household access to firearms in Colorado: results of a case-control study. J Adolesc Health 2000;26:157–63.
15. Bennett DS. Depression among children with chronic medical problems: a meta-analysis. J Pediatr Psychol 1994;19:149–69.
16. American Psychiatric Association. Diagnostic and statistical manual of mental disorders: DSM-IV-TR. 4th ed., text revision. Washington, DC: APA; 2000.
17. Jellinek MS, Snyder JB. Depression and suicide in children and adolescents. Pediatr Rev 1998;19:255–64.
18. Silverman JG, Raj A, Mucci LA, Hathaway JE. Dating violence against adolescent girls and associated substance use, unhealthy weight control, sexual risk behavior, pregnancy, and suicidality. JAMA 2001;286:572–9.
19. U.S. Department of Health and Human Services. The Surgeon General's call to action to prevent suicide. Washington, DC: USDHHS; 1999. Available at: http://www.surgeongeneral.gov/library/calltoaction/calltoaction.pdf. Retrieved October 17, 2002.
20. Russell ST, Joyner K. Adolescent sexual orientation and suicide risk: evidence from a national study. Am J Public Health 2001;91:1276–81.
21. Suicide and suicide attempts in adolescents. Committee on Adolescence. American Academy of Pediatrics. Pediatrics 2000;105:871–4.
22. Bayatpour M, Wells RD, Holford S. Physical and sexual abuse as predictors of substance use and suicide among pregnant teenagers. J Adolesc Health 1992;13:128–32.
23. Koniak-Griffin D, Lesser J. The impact of childhood maltreatment of young mothers' violent behavior toward themselves and others. J Pediatr Nurs 1996;11:300–8.
24. Stack S. New microlevel data on the impact of divorce on suicide, 1959–1980: a test of two theories. J Marriage Fam 1990;52:119–27.
25. Barnet B, Joffe A, Doggan AK, Wilson MD, Repke JT. Depressive symptoms, stress, and social support in pregnant and postpartum adolescents. Arch Pediatr Adolesc Med 1996;150:64–9.
26. Berman AL, Jobes DA. Adolescent suicide: assessment and intervention. Washington, DC: American Psychological Association; 1991.
27. Tishler CL. Adolescent suicide: assessment of risk, prevention, and treatment. Adolesc Med 1992;3:51–60.
28. Miller MC, Jacobs DG, Gutheil TG. Talisman or taboo: the controversy of the suicide-prevention contract. Harv Rev Psychiatry 1998;6:78–87.

Resources

ACOG Resources

American College of Obstetricians and Gynecologists. Depression. ACOG Patient Education Pamphlet AP106. Washington, DC: ACOG; 1999.

American College of Obstetricians and Gynecologists. Postpartum depression. ACOG Patient Education Pamphlet AP091. Washington, DC: ACOG; 1999.

American College of Obstetricians and Gynecologists. Tool kit for teen care. Washington, DC: ACOG; 2003.

Dell DL. Depression in women. Clin Updat Womens Health Care 2002;1(2):1–81.

OTHER RESOURCES

The following lists are for information purposes only. Referral to these sources and web sites does not imply the endorsement of ACOG. These lists are not meant to be comprehensive. The exclusion of a source or web site does not reflect the quality of that source or web site. Please note that web sites are subject to change without notice.

American Academy of Child and Adolescent Psychiatry
3615 Wisconsin Avenue NW
Washington, DC 20016-3007
Tel: (202) 966-7300
Fax: (202) 966-2891
Web: www.aacap.org

American Academy of Family Physicians
11400 Tomahawk Creek Parkway
Leawood, KS 66211-2672
Tel: (913) 906-6000
Web: www.aafp.org

American Academy of Pediatrics
141 Northwest Point Boulevard
Elk Grove Village, IL 60007-1098
Tel: (847) 434-4000
Fax: (847) 434-8000
Web: www.aap.org

American Association of Suicidology
4201 Connecticut Avenue NW, Suite 408
Washington, DC 20008
Tel: (202) 237-2280
Fax: (202) 237-2282
Web: www.suicidology.org

American Psychiatric Association
1400 K Street NW
Washington, DC 20005
Tel: 888-357-7924
Fax: (202) 682-6850
Web: www.psych.org

American Psychological Association
750 First Street NE
Washington, DC 20002-4242
Tel: 800-374-2721; (202) 336-5510
Web: www.apa.org

The Center for Mental Health Services
PO Box 42490
Washington, DC 20015
Tel: 800-789-2647
Fax: (301) 984-8796
Web: www.mentalhealth.org

The Society for Adolescent Medicine
1916 NW Copper Oaks Circle
Blue Springs, MO 64015
Tel: (816) 224-8010
Web: www.adolescenthealth.org

RESOURCES FOR YOUR PATIENTS

AWARE Foundation
1015 Chestnut Street, Suite 1225
Philadelphia, PA 19107-4302
Tel: (215) 955-9847
Web: www.awarefoundation.org

Center for Young Women's Health
Children's Hospital
333 Longwood Avenue, 5th floor
Boston, MA 02115
Tel: (617) 355-CYWH (2994)
Fax: (617) 232-3136
Web: www.youngwomenshealth.org

Go Ask Alice! (by Columbia University Health Education Program)
Lerner Hall
2920 Broadway, 7th Floor
MC 2608
New York, NY 10027
Tel: (212) 854-5453
Fax: (212) 854-8949
Web: www.goaskalice.columbia.edu

National Women's Health Information Center (by DHHS Office on Women's Health)
8550 Arlington Boulevard, Suite 300
Fairfax, VA 22031
Tel: 800-994-WOMAN
Web: www.4woman.org; www.4girls.gov

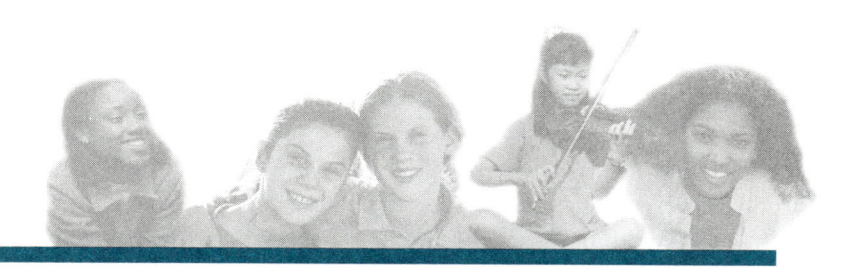

Appendix A

Comprehensive Reproductive Health Services for Adolescents*

Adolescence is a time of psychosocial, cognitive, and physical development as young people make the transition from childhood to adulthood. This transition includes sexual development and often entails behaviors that put young women at risk for pregnancy and sexually transmitted diseases. Guidance from a physician, as well as needed reproductive health screening and care, can greatly facilitate young people's healthy transition to adulthood.

Health care professionals have an obligation to provide the best possible care to respond to the needs of their adolescent patients. This care should, at a minimum, include comprehensive reproductive health services, such as sexuality education, counseling, mental health assessment, diagnosis and treatment regarding pubertal development, access to contraceptives and abortion, pregnancy-related care, prenatal and delivery care, and diagnosis and treatment of sexually transmitted diseases. Every effort should be made to include male partners in such services and counseling.

Comprehensive services may be delivered to adolescents in a variety of sites, including schools, physician offices, and community-based and other health care facilities. Legal barriers that restrict the freedom of health care practitioners to provide these services should be removed. Institutional policies should be developed to require practitioners with views on confidentiality that restrict the provision of services to a minor to refer the patient to another practitioner.

Because the involvement of a concerned adult can contribute to the health and success of an adolescent, policies in health care settings should encourage and facilitate communication between a minor and her parent(s), when appropriate. However, concerns about confidentiality, as well as economic considerations, can be significant barriers to reproductive health care for some adolescents. The potential health risks to adolescents if they are unable to obtain reproductive health services are so compelling that legal barriers and deference to parental involvement should not stand in the way of needed health care for patients who request confidentiality. Therefore, laws and regulations that are unduly restrictive of adolescents' confidential access to reproductive health care should be revised. Institutional proce-

---

*American College of Obstetricians and Gynecologists. Patient care. In: Guidelines for women's health care. 2nd ed. Washington: DC: ACOG; 2002. p. 145–6.

dures that safeguard the rights of their adolescent patients, including confidentiality during initial and subsequent visits and in billing, should be established.

Billing mechanisms for services and procedures for insurance and other third-party reimbursement should ensure adolescent confidentiality. When these mechanisms and procedures compromise a patient's request for confidentiality, policies should be implemented allowing payment alternatives such as reduced fees, sliding scales, and timed installment payments and patient referral to a practice or agency where subsidized care is offered or both.

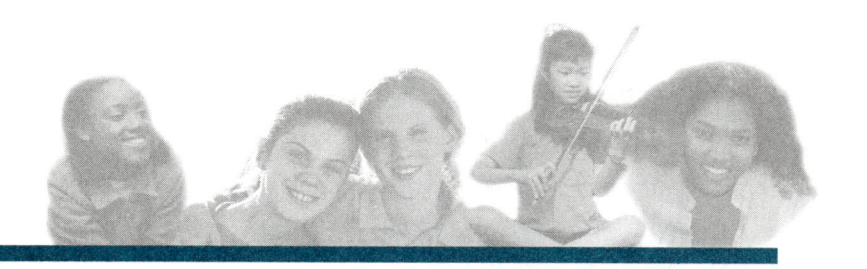

Appendix B

Sexuality Education*

The American College of Obstetricians and Gynecologists supports the inclusion of age-appropriate sexuality education from kindergarten through 12th grade as an integral part of comprehensive health education in schools and communities. The American College of Obstetricians and Gynecologists encourages its members to advocate for and participate in such education.

Efforts to encourage young people to delay becoming sexually active are components of almost all sexuality education programs. These programs typically are described as "abstinence-only," "abstinence-based," "abstinence-plus," and "abstinence-centered." One particular form of "abstinence-only" education is characterized by a definition of abstinence included in recent federal welfare reform law that narrowly describes its contents and purposes. This federal law, along with other factors, has contributed to a growing emphasis by some on limiting sexuality education so as to exclude accurate instruction about contraception, abortion, and sexual orientation. A recent report indicates that as of 1999, 4 in 10 sexuality education teachers in secondary public schools either teach that birth control and condoms are ineffective means of preventing pregnancy and STDs or do not cover birth control or condoms at all. Abstinence "based/plus/centered" programs, by contrast, not only promote abstinence but also incorporate reproductive health information, including both the risks and benefits of various methods of contraception, STD prevention, and forms of sexual expression alternative to intercourse.

Sexuality education programs, in general, have not been well evaluated. In particular, the impact on behavior of "abstinence-only" programs has not yet been documented through appropriate research. However, some "abstinence-based" programs that include positive messages and promote contraceptive use among those who are sexually active have shown modest success in delaying the initiation of sexual activity and increasing the use of contra-

---

*American College of Obstetricians and Gynecologists. Patient care. In: Guidelines for women's health care. 2nd ed. Washington: DC: ACOG; 2002. p. 148–50.

ception. Communities planning appropriate sexuality education for adolescents should consider the following points which are supported by ACOG:

- Parental involvement in their child(ren)'s sexuality education
- The goal of promoting healthy lifestyles for adolescents and their families. This includes the following objectives:
  - Promote abstinence from sexual intercourse as the preferred responsible behavior for adolescents
  - Increase effective use of contraceptives, including latex condoms, by sexually active adolescents
  - Support increased availability of confidential reproductive health services, including family planning and services for the prevention, diagnosis, and/or treatment of STDs
- All sexuality education programs should provide scientifically accurate information about sexuality, STDs, contraception, and preventive health care
- Ongoing rigorous evaluation of the effectiveness of a variety of forms of sexuality education in terms of their effect on sexual behavior, as well as unintended pregnancy and abortion rates

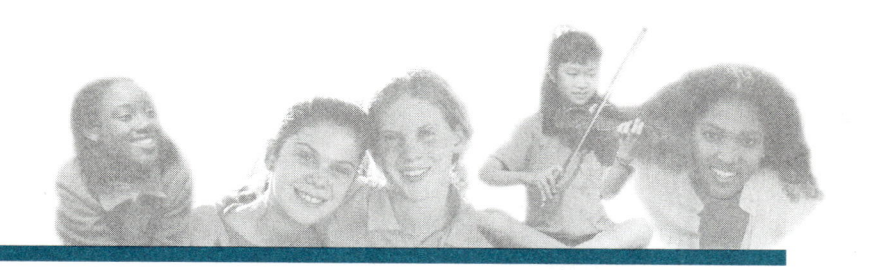

Index

Note: Page numbers followed by the letters *f* and *t* indicate figures and tables, respectively.

A

Abortion, 16, 25, 29–30
Abstinence, 16, in sexuality education, 109–110
Abuse
  screening for, 18–19
  and suicide risk, 95, 98, 99
Acne, oral contraceptives and, 40–41
Acquired immunodeficiency syndrome (AIDS), rates of, 55. *See also* Human immunodeficiency virus
Adenocarcinoma, oral contraceptives and, 43
Adolescent(s)
  development of, 3–5
    cognitive, 4–5
    psychosocial, 4–5
    sexual, 4
  as emancipated minors, 29
  health guidance for, 8–9
  health risks to, 1, 3, 27
  legal status of, 27
  as mature minors, 25, 29
  sexually active. *See* Sexually active adolescents
Adolescent pregnancy
  rates of, 16, 46, 55
  and suicide risk, 99
Adoption, 16
African Americans, sexual development of, 4
Age
  and blood pressure, 12*f*
  and body mass index, 15*f*
  and stature, 10*f*
AIDS. *See* Acquired immunodeficiency syndrome
Alcohol use, screening for, 14–16
Amenorrhea
  anorexia nervosa and, 86
  female athlete triad and, 90
  oral contraceptives and, 44

Anemia, iron deficiency, oral contraceptives and, 40
Anorexia nervosa, 81, 83, 84–86
  definition of, 84
  differential diagnosis of, 85
  health consequences of, 86
  history and physical examination for, 84–85
  screening for, 12–14
  treatment of, 85–86
Anovulation, oral contraceptives and, 41
Antiphospholipid antibodies, oral contraceptives and, 44
Aspiration pneumonia, bulimia nervosa and, 88

B

Benign breast disease, oral contraceptives and, 40
Binge eating disorder, 81, 83, 89
  definition of, 89
  health consequences of, 89
  history and physical examination for, 89
  treatment of, 89
Birth control pills. *See* Oral contraceptives
Blood pressure
  classification of, 9–11
  screening for, 9–11
BMI. *See* Body mass index
Body image
  and eating disorders, 83
  media and, 8
Body mass index (BMI)
  by age, 15*f*
  anorexia nervosa and, 85
  calculation of, 12, 13*f*
  and obesity, 14
Body size, and blood pressure, 9, 12*f*

Bone mineral density
  anorexia nervosa and, 86
  female athlete triad and, 90
  oral contraceptives and, 41
Breakthrough bleeding, oral contraceptives and, 45
Breast budding, 4
Breast cancer, oral contraceptives and, 43
Breast disease, benign, oral contraceptives and, 40
Breast tenderness, oral contraceptives and, 45
Bulimia nervosa, 81, 83, 86–88
  definition of, 86–87
  health consequences of, 88
  history and physical examination for, 88
  screening for, 12–14
  treatment of, 88

C

Cancer
  condoms and, 56
  oral contraceptives and, 41, 42–43
Cardiomyopathy, bulimia nervosa and, 88
Cardiovascular disease, oral contraceptives and, 42
Cathartic colon, bulimia nervosa and, 88
Cerebrovascular disease, oral contraceptives and, 42
Cervical cancer, condoms and, 56
Cervical intraepithelial neoplasia (CIN), oral contraceptives and, 43
Cervical neoplasia, oral contraceptives and, 43
Chancroid, prevention of transmission of, condoms and, 56
Childhood immunization schedule, 21*f*
Chlamydia
  geographic variation in cases of, 71
  prevention of transmission of, 56
  rates of, 55

Chlamydia *(continued)*
  reported cases of, 71
  screening for, 17, 69–75
    candidates for, 72
    methods of, 74t
    urine tests, 73–74
  sexual assault and, 74–75
Cholesterol, screening for, 11–12
Cigarette smoking
  and oral contraceptive use, 42
  screening for, 14
CIN. *See* Cervical intraepithelial neoplasia
Cognitive development, 4–5
Comprehensive reproductive health services, 107–108
Condoms, 53–59
  availability of, 53, 58–59
  effectiveness of, 55–56
  failure rates of, 56
  female, 56
  natural membrane, 56
  popularity of, 39, 57
  use of
    barriers to, 53, 58–59
    in conjunction with other contraceptive methods, 56, 57
    correct and consistent, 57
    factors affecting, 57
Confidentiality, 5, 25–33
  addressing, 28
  barriers to, 27
  contraceptives and, 39–40
  economics and, 27, 33
  legal issues involving, 28–30
  in office visits, 30–33, 30t
  parents and, 25, 28, 30, 30t, 31
Consent
  by adolescents, 28–30
  by parents, 25, 27
Contraception, 16
  choice of, 39
  condoms, 53–59
  and confidentiality, 39–40
  effectiveness of, 56
  failure rates of, 56
  long-term, refusal of, 63–66
  oral contraceptives, 37–47
  postpartum, 46
  rate of use of, 39
Coronary heart disease, risk of developing, 11

D

Date rape, 18
Death, among adolescents, causes of, 3
Delayed fertility, oral contraceptives and, 44

Depression
  and binge eating disorder, 89
  screening for, 18
  and suicide risk, 18, 99–100
Diastolic blood pressure, 9–11, 12f
Dietary habits, 8
Diphtheria, tetanus, pertussis vaccine, 21f
Diuretics, and bulimia nervosa, 86, 88
Divorce, and suicide risk, 99
Drug overdose, and suicide, 98
Drug use, screening for, 14–16
Dysmenorrhea, oral contraceptives and, 40

E

Eating disorders, 81–91. *See also specific disorders*
  etiology of, 83
  presentations of, 84
  prevention of, 91
  screening for, 12–14, 84
Economics, and confidentiality, 27, 33
Ectopic pregnancy, oral contraceptives and, 41
Egocentrism, 4–5
Emancipated minors, 29
Embolism, oral contraceptives and, 41–42
Emergency care, consent and, 29
Emergency contraception pills, 16, 39
Endocervical specimen tests, for sexually transmitted diseases, 69
Endometrial cancer, oral contraceptives and, 41, 42
Esophageal rupture, bulimia nervosa and, 88
Esophagitis, bulimia nervosa and, 88
Estrogen
  in oral contraceptives
    and breakthrough bleeding, 45
    and thromboembolism, 41–42
  and sexual development, 4
Exercise
  female athlete triad and, 90
  promotion of, 8

F

Factor V Leiden, and thromboembolism, 42
Female athlete triad, 81, 83, 90–91
  definition of, 90
  health consequences of, 90–91
  history and physical examination for, 90
  treatment of, 90
Female condom, 56
Fertility, delayed, oral contraceptives and, 44
Firearms, and suicide, 95, 98
Functional ovarian cysts, oral contraceptives and, 40

G

GAPS. *See* Guidelines for Adolescent Preventive Services
Gender, and suicide risk, 95, 97
Genital herpes, prevention of transmission of, 56
Gonorrhea
  geographic variation in cases of, 71
  prevention of transmission of, 56
  rates of, 55
  reported cases of, 71
  screening for, 17, 69–75
    candidates for, 72
    methods of, 74t
    urine tests, 73–74
  sexual assault and, 74–75
Guidelines for Adolescent Preventive Services (GAPS), 6
Guns, and suicide, 95, 98

H

Haemophilus influenzae Type b vaccine, 21f
Hanging, and suicide, 98
Headaches, oral contraceptives and, 44, 45
Health care visits, 107–108
  annual, 1, 6
  confidentiality in, 30–33, 30t
  initial, 1, 5
Health guidance, 1, 6–9
  for adolescents, 8–9
  for parents, 7–8
Height
  and blood pressure, 9, 12f
  and body mass index, 13f
  oral contraceptives and, 44
  during sexual development, 4
Hepatitis A immunization, 20, 21f
Hepatitis B immunization, 20, 21f
Herpes, genital, prevention of transmission of, 56
High-normal blood pressure, 9
HIV. *See* Human immunodeficiency virus
Human immunodeficiency virus (HIV). *See also* Acquired immunodeficiency syndrome
  prevention of transmission of, 56
  screening for, 17–18
Human papillomavirus
  oral contraceptives and, 43
  prevention of transmission of, 56
Hyperlipidemia, risk of developing, 11
Hypertension
  classification of, 9–11
  oral contraceptives and, 42, 44
Hypertriglyceridemia, oral contraceptives and, 44

Index

Hypokalemia, bulimia nervosa and, 88
Hypomagnesemia, bulimia nervosa and, 88
Hypophosphatemia, bulimia nervosa and, 88

I

Immunizations, 19–20, 21f
Implantable contraceptives
　popularity of, 39
　refusal of, 63–66
Influenza vaccine, 21f
Injectable contraceptives
　popularity of, 39
　refusal of, 63–66
Injury(ies), prevention of, 9
Insurance
　and confidentiality, 33
　and oral contraceptives, 40
Invulnerability, feelings of, 4–5
Iron deficiency anemia, oral contraceptives and, 40

J

Judicial bypass, for abortion without parental consent, 29–30

L

Laboratory results, confidentiality and, 31
Lactation, oral contraceptives and, 46
Latex condoms. *See* Condoms
Laxatives, and bulimia nervosa, 86, 88
Legal issues
　involving confidentiality, 28–30
　involving long-term contraception, 65–66
　involving parental consent, 27
　involving sexual assault, 74–75
Ligase chain reaction tests, for sexually transmitted diseases, 69, 73, 74t
Long-term contraception, refusal of, 63–66

M

Mallory-Weiss lesions, bulimia nervosa and, 88
Malnutrition, health consequences of, 86
Mature minor, 25, 29
Measles–mumps–rubella vaccine, 20, 21f
Media
　and body image, 8
　suicide coverage in, 99
Medicaid, 27
Menarche, 4
Menstrual irregularity
　anorexia nervosa and, 86
　female athlete triad and, 90
　oral contraceptives and, 40, 41, 44, 45

Migraine headaches, oral contraceptives and, 44
Minors. *See* Adolescent(s)
Mortality, among adolescents, causes of, 3
Myocardial infarction, oral contraceptives and, 42

N

National Strategy for Suicide Prevention, 97
Natural membrane condoms, 56
Nausea, oral contraceptives and, 45
Nicotine therapy, 14
No-suicide contracts, 101
Norethindrone mini-pills, 46
Nucleic acid amplification technique tests, for sexually transmitted diseases, 69, 73, 74t
Nutrition, 8

O

Obesity
　binge eating disorder and, 89
　screening for, 12–14
OCs. *See* Oral contraceptives
Oligomenorrhea
　female athlete triad and, 90
　oral contraceptives and, 44
Oral contraceptives (OCs), 16, 37–47
　benefits of, 37, 40–41
　complications and side effects of, 37, 41–45
　contraindications to, 37, 44
　correct and consistent use of, 46
　costs of, 40
　deterrents to use of, 37, 41–44
　discontinuation of use, 44–45
　failure rate of, 39
　initial visit for, 37, 39
　popularity of, 39
　postpartum use of, 46
　sexually transmitted diseases and, 45
Osteoporosis, female athlete triad and, 90
Ovarian cancer, oral contraceptives and, 41, 42

P

Pancreatitis, bulimia nervosa and, 88
Pap test, initial, 1, 5
Paralytic ileus, bulimia nervosa and, 88
Parent(s)
　and confidentiality, 25, 28, 30, 30t, 31
　consent of, 25, 27
　health guidance for, 7–8
　and long-term contraception, 65–66
Payment, and confidentiality, 33

Pelvic examination
　annual, 6
　initial, 1, 5
　and sexually transmitted disease screening, 72
Pelvic inflammatory disease (PID), oral contraceptives and, 41
Physical activity, 8
Physical examination, 6
　for anorexia nervosa, 84–85
　for binge eating disorder, 89
　for bulimia nervosa, 88
　confidentiality and, 31
　for female athlete triad, 90
PID. *See* Pelvic inflammatory disease
Pneumococcal vaccine, 21f
Pneumomediastinum, bulimia nervosa and, 88
Poisoning, and suicide, 95, 98
Polycystic ovary syndrome
　binge eating disorder and, 89
　bulimia nervosa and, 88
Postpartum use, of oral contraceptives, 46
Pregnancy. *See also* Adolescent pregnancy
　ectopic, oral contraceptives and, 41
　prevention of. *See* Contraception
　while using oral contraceptives, 45
Preventive primary health care, 1–20
Primary health care, 1–20
Progestogens, in oral contraceptives, and thromboembolism, 42
Psychosocial development, 4–5
Puberty, duration of, 4
Purging bulimia, 86

R

Race/ethnicity, and suicide risk, 95, 97
Rape, date, 18
Renal disease, oral contraceptives and, 44

S

School(s)
　condom availability in, 58
　sexuality education programs in, 109–110
School performance, assessment of, 19
Screening(s), 1, 9–19
　for abuse, 18–19
　for alcohol use, 14–16
　for blood pressure, 9–11
　for chlamydia, 69–75
　for cholesterol, 11–12
　for depression, 18
　for drug use, 14–16
　for eating disorders, 12–14, 84
　for gonorrhea, 69–75
　for human immunodeficiency virus, 17–18

Screening(s) *(continued)*
  for sexually active adolescents, 1, 16–17
  for sexually transmitted diseases, 1, 6, 17, 69–75
  for tobacco use, 14
  for tuberculosis, 19
Selective serotonin reuptake inhibitors (SSRIs)
  for anorexia nervosa, 86
  for binge eating disorder, 89
Self-esteem, 8
Sexual activity, increase in, condom availability and, 58–59
Sexual assault, and sexually transmitted diseases, 74–75
Sexual development, 4, premature, 4
Sexuality education programs, 109–110
Sexually active adolescents
  annual health care visit of, 6
  condom availability to, 58–59
  initial health care visit of, 5
  initiation of sexual activity, 55
  responsible behavior of, 8–9
  screenings for, 1, 16–17
Sexually transmitted diseases (STDs). *See also specific sexually transmitted diseases*
  condoms and, 53
  oral contraceptives and, 45
  protection against, 16, 55–56
  rates of, 55, 71
  screenings for, 1, 6, 17, 69–75
  sexual assault and, 74–75

Smoking
  and oral contraceptive use, 42
  screening for, 14
SSRIs. *See* Selective serotonin reuptake inhibitors
Stature. *See* Height
STDs. *See* Sexually transmitted diseases
Stress, and suicide risk, 98–99
Stunted growth, oral contraceptives and, 44
Substance abuse, screening for, 14–16
Suffocation, and suicide, 98
Suicide
  depression and, 18, 99–100
  methods of, 95, 98
  prevention of, 95–102, 100–101
  rate of, 95, 97
  risk assessment of, 100–101
  risk factors for, 95, 98–100
Syphilis
  prevention of transmission of, 56
  screening for, 17
Systemic lupus erythematosus, oral contraceptives and, 44
Systolic blood pressure, 9–11, 12*f*

T

Tetanus–diphtheria vaccine, 20, 21*f*
Thelarche, 4

Thromboembolism, oral contraceptives and, 41–42
Tobacco use
  and oral contraceptives use, 42
  screening for, 14
Toxic shock syndrome, oral contraceptives and, 41
Treatment plans, confidentiality and, 31
Tuberculosis, screening for, 19
2001 Youth Risk Behavior Surveillance Report, 3

U

Urine screening, for sexually transmitted diseases, 69, 73–74

V

Vaccinations, 19–20, 21*f*
Varicella vaccine, 20, 21*f*
Venous thrombosis, oral contraceptives and, 41–42
Vomiting, bulimia nervosa and, 86, 88

W

Weight
  and body mass index, 13*f*
  oral contraceptives and, 44–45
Withdrawal bleeding, oral contraceptives and, 44, 45